The Muscle & Hustle Method

ED DJAFER

ISBN: 1723134686
ISBN-13: 9781723134685

DEDICATION

I dedicate this book to my beautiful wife to be Helen, and my boy Jaiden. You've backed me and been there for me through thick and thin, and through all the years of HUSTLE, even at times when I doubted myself. I thank you for all your love and support. Without which, none of this would have been possible.

Thank you for making my dreams come true.

You are my world!

CONTENTS

ACKNOWLEDGMENTS

Thank you to my coach Tim Drummond for helping me to take big action. This book would have still been a dream sitting in my head if it wasn't for your accountability and holding my feet to the fire at times.

Thank you to Phil Hawksworth for helping me to pull out every ounce of information from all four corners of my brain and speed up the process of getting the words from my mind down on paper.

Thank you to the thousands of clients that I've had the opportunity to work with over the years, and for all your support. Without you this book wouldn't have been possible.

1 INTRODUCTION

"Enough is enough!
I need to do something about this.
Now!".

I'd just got back from holiday and was looking at the photos of myself on the beach. I felt sick to my stomach seeing the man boobs and flabby sides hanging over. This isn't who I wanted to be. I don't want to look like this. I don't want to live my life feeling like this.

Trudging along, living a mediocre life. I had greater aspirations than this, and damnit I was going to make it happen.

Let's Begin...

It all started for me when I was 14 years old. I got my first set of weights for my birthday. Obviously going through my teens, my body was changing, and I was becoming aware and self-conscious of how my body was looking. Hormones are naturally up and down at that age as you're going through puberty. That's when I started to develop man boobs.

That's not abnormal for teenage boys. It's usually a phase and you typically grow out of it in a year or two. Not me, I got through my teens, going into my twenties and the man boobs weren't disappearing. They didn't go anywhere – if anything they were getting worse as I got older - I still had man boobs in to my twenties and I **hated** the way I looked.

By this point in my life I was going out more, being more social with friends from work. No longer wearing a school uniform, I was extremely self-conscious of what I wore and would avoid anything tight or fitted. If it showed off my body shape, it wasn't in my wardrobe.

Dealing with my body issues was affecting my confidence, my self-esteem, and it was holding me back from coming out of my shell, having fun, and meeting women. I simply wasn't comfortable in my body. I was always shy anyway, and not having confidence in my body certainly didn't make things any easier. I'd avoid going out with people I didn't know, would never approach people I wasn't already friends with, and was always the one sat in the corner quietly, waiting for someone to come and talk to me.

There came I point that I realised that I wasn't the person I wanted to be. This might sound funny now that I'm older, but back then I would see people on TV that I looked up to. I used to be really into WWE wrestling and I would see those guys who looked great, had a lot of charisma and character. They were superstars.

Deep down inside, that's who I wanted to be. Not necessarily such an extrovert or outgoing kind of guy, just someone who had that confidence and certainty in their self. That feeling of being comfortable in your own skin and not afraid to show who you are. That's really all I wanted.

As I got into my twenties I knew that things had to change. If you're familiar with me, you might have seen that picture where I'm on holiday on the beach; I've got a flabby belly and man boobs – that was really the turning point for me. Looking at those holiday photos when I was back home, I felt sick to my stomach. I couldn't go on like this. I said enough was enough, I don't want to be that person anymore.

When I was a kid, I never had issues with my body or the way I looked, but all through my teenage years, my confidence started dropping and that was affecting my life in other areas. It was impacting the decisions I was making and the opportunities that I took in my studies and what I wanted to do with my life as I became an adult and moved into employment. My lack of confidence was holding me back from becoming the man I wanted to become.

I followed the example of my parents. Not that they were a bad example to follow, but it wasn't truly the path that I wanted to follow. In terms of career, business, and what I want to do with my life; I wanted to be my own man, to follow my own path. Insecurity was holding me back from doing that. I would always second guess myself, and could never rid myself of that voice in the back of my head saying I wasn't good enough, or who was I to do that?

My parents have always taught me to be very cautious. To play within my comfort zone. Of course, it's what parents do. They're just trying to protect their kids, which obviously is not a bad thing. However, for me, I always wanted to have the confidence to push out of my comfort zone and be my own person. To do more with my life than perhaps would have been possible just following the safe, comfortable path that my life trajectory was set on.

When I was 21 years old, after that beach holiday, I said that enough was enough. I wanted to change my body, I wanted to become a person who is comfortable in their own skin. To be confident in pursuing the path I wanted to be on and build the kind of life I wanted to live. I knew once I had confidence in myself, everything else would start to fall in to place. Thankfully I realised that early on. My own confidence was the key to achieve the things I wanted to do in business, in my relationships, and in the rest of my life.

At no point was it an easy journey. There was a lot of trial and error along the way. It all began when I started working out at home. I got some weights for my 14th birthday, which had been sitting around for years collecting dust, so I started using them at home. I had used them on and off over the previous years, and when I was giving them a go, I did see some positive results, but had never really stuck to it.

Being very on and off was a pattern throughout my teenage years. Other things would take priority and I wasn't making exercise a part of my life on a permanent basis. I'd train for a few weeks, feel my biceps were getting a bit bigger and stronger, which would make me feel good and build a little confidence; but then I'd stop and get distracted by something else.

It was only when I could see I was losing the results that I would get back into it. There was a lot of stopping and starting there at the beginning. This went on until I finally made that commitment when I was about 21 years old. That was the turning point, when I saw that photo of me on holiday. I'd already been training a little bit on and off, but this time it was different. That was the time that I made the commitment to transform. Not just 'to train', but to **transform** my body.

5

I immersed myself into fitness; learning everything I could about training, about diet and nutrition. I tried every diet going, so I know from experience that they don't work. I would lose weight and put weight back on. There was a lot of yo-yoing up and down, similar to the struggles that most people go through when it comes to weight loss or body transformation. One step forwards, and then one step back.

Instead of seeing it as a lifestyle, many – and this included me for years - see it as temporary fix to lose 10lbs. You must ask yourself; what happens beyond that?

The thing that made the difference for me was that I started to take a long-term view and see it as a lifestyle. I wanted to make it a permanent part of my lifestyle, instead of another quick fix. I wanted to make it part of who I was. I started looking for ways that I could incorporate it into my life. At first, I became very obsessive. I was reading all the bodybuilding magazines, reading about fitness online, falling for all the marketing from supplement companies telling me I could get shredded with some pill or potion for only £39.95.

I literally spent thousands of pounds on supplements. It's a powerful industry and the marketing is very clever when it comes to convincing desperate young men to part with their money. What I failed to see at the time was that it is the basics that get you results. Good nutrition, training hard and consistently, and sticking with it for an extended period, is what brings results. Not some mass gainer product or weight loss supplement. Sure, they can help, if used correctly. But as the name suggests, they are there to supplement and assist with the process, not to replace a chunk of your diet, or do the work for you. It's simply about being consistent and putting in the work over time.

I guess the difference between myself and others. Or myself at 21 versus myself in the years earlier, was that I was willing to try things, often fail, but not quit. Every time I failed, I didn't see it as a failure, it was just another part of the learning curve, another part of the journey. Every failure was a stepping stone closer to the end I wanted.

For many people, when they fail, especially when they fail repeatedly; it stops them. They quit persevering and resign themselves to settling for less than they'd ideally want.

I wasn't willing to give in. I was very resilient and determined. If I failed, I would try another way, and if that failed, I would find another way again.

I'm a tenacious little fucker at times! You never stop learning on this journey. Whether that's in fitness, in business, or just in life; you never stop learning. There's always going to be failure along the way. There will always be struggles, but that's part of the fun.

There's always progress that can be made, but you're also always going to face sticking points and obstacles. What you soon realise is that the obstacles are not there to stop you, they're there to push you a little harder. For you to overcome, and become better, become stronger. The more times you fail, the more obstacles you get through, the better and stronger you will be. Each obstacle is an opportunity for growth. If you keep growing, you will eventually overcome anything that is in your way.

On this journey of life, whether in fitness, business, or life generally; you're always going to struggle. There are always obstacles and failures along the way. There's always something else to overcome and challenge you, and that means you're always learning along the way. It never ends. As soon as you overcome one barrier, you are faced with another.

My advice would be to embrace the failures. Fail as many times as you possibly can. You never lose in life, you either win, or you learn. 'Failure' is not a bad thing. In fact, it's a good thing. It's not the end, it's just part of the process. It's how we grow as people, as entrepreneurs, and as men.

My journey started with learning how to transform my body. After overcoming the struggles, I had there, I was able to take that learning; the process and some of the lessons I learnt from health and fitness and apply them to other areas of my life. Some of the things I learnt in my body transformation were responsible for helping me to build a successful coaching business, which brings me to where I am now. Helping other people.

I got in to coaching because I found something that I love to do, that made me excited to get up in the morning and go to work. Previously, I was stuck in a job which had inconsistent hours, working for somebody else, and doing a job where day to day I didn't enjoy the work. Being told what to do wasn't something I was comfortable with. I wanted to be my own boss and be in control of my own life. I didn't want anyone else having that hold over me.

After I'd been through my physical transformation and developed a much greater level of confidence than I previously had, I made the decision to leave my regular, secure job. To take a risk, gamble, and back myself following my passion to get into the fitness industry.

It started with me personal training a few friends. My friends started getting great results in their transformations and soon other people were asking me to train them too. After I decided that I was leaving my job I went and became a Personal Trainer, got myself qualified and followed the same process of learning as before. Going through the same kinds of struggles, the same failures as when I was doing my body transformation.

None of that mattered. I was determined to leave my regular day job behind to pursue my dreams. That meant me having to go back into studying, which I had to do in my spare time while also having a full-time job to support myself. The study was like another full-time job, learning not only how to become a Personal Trainer, but also how to build a business for myself.

I immersed myself in it. Taking what I'd learnt from my own transformation over the previous years, I already knew a lot. I knew what it took to create a body transformation, after being in the trenches and doing it myself. Even though I knew by that point what to eat and how to train, studying to become certified was a totally different ball game. I had to learn every bone in the body, how the heart and lungs work; all kinds of stuff that I don't really use in my everyday business. It just had to be done to pursue this dream of becoming a personal trainer and getting all the certifications in order. The funny thing is, people don't care about what qualifications you have as long as you can demonstrate how much you care, and you can get them the results they want. My first business coach once told me "People don't care about how much you know, until they know how much you care". In all my years in the fitness industry, not one client has ever asked to see my certificates.

There were a lot of struggles early on. This was my first business, I was a quiet, naturally shy person and I had to learn a lot of things through trial and error, just like when I was transforming my physique. It took me a while to get on my feet and figure out how to consistently get clients, even though I was getting superb results with the ones who did come on board.

I did Personal Training for 10 years, loved it, and worked with thousands of clients over those years. Becoming quite well known for my 30-minute express workouts. Being able to get a great workout done in a short period of time and getting great results for the busy executives I worked with. I even prepped a client for a fitness show where she took a couple of medals, still with just half hour workouts a few times per week. I'll tell you more about her story and the workouts a little later.

These short, intense workouts are ideal for the kind of people I work with now. Busy guys who want to get in and out of the gym, not spending hours of time on this. Just get in, get their workout done, and get on with the rest of their day.

After 10 years of Personal Training, I decided that it was time to leave a good job behind, for something even greater. I was at a point where I was in my comfort zone again. I'm the kind of person as an entrepreneur who always wants to be pushing, to do more and better myself. To do that, I had to be prepared to leave behind what was comfortable, even leave behind what is great, to take a gamble and back myself to achieve something even greater. That's how I got into coaching.

I left behind the successful Personal Training business to become a Health and Performance Coach. To help busy, male entrepreneurs and business owners not only to transform their body, but to use that journey, the process; and apply it to the rest of their life. Their business, relationships, and everything else that is important.

I help entrepreneurs not only become healthier and fitter, but I also help them to get a return on their investment and improve their business, using some of the same principles we use in transforming our body. The same discipline and effort. The success habits that we build up through our commitment to building a great physique.

That's what you can expect in this book, I will be sharing how to apply the principles I have used to transform my own and my client's bodies. How you can take these same principles and success habits and apply them in your business.

There are 3 common things that you need to succeed in both body and business. The 3 elements of the 'Muscle & Hustle' method are Build, Systemise, and Vision.

The first component, build. Whether we are building a body or building a business; the principles are the same. You must put in the work, it takes consistent effort to get things off the ground. You must be prepared to put in the reps and fail, to learn, and overcome challenges, rather than letting them stop you.

Once you get past that resistance, you get to a point where you can systemise things. In our health and body, the systemisation is the daily habits that you adopt. Consistently eating a well-balanced diet, working out, and living a healthy lifestyle become habits. They become part of your lifestyle, just like running your business is part of your lifestyle. When you've been doing it long enough, you can do it in your sleep. It runs almost on autopilot.

In business you automate and outsource things, so your business runs without you having to put in so much effort. To a point where you don't even have to be there. When you build the healthy habits, the same applies to your body. Both body and business can run on autopilot, without you having to put in consistent mental effort.

At this stage you get to the third component; vision. Having a bigger picture view of why you're doing what you're doing. Initially, your goal might be to lose 10lbs, but now we start to see the bigger vision. What will losing 10lbs do for you? How will it benefit your life? Where do you go next? What happens when we attain our goals? What's next?

We start to see the bigger picture things; like being healthier will give us more time on this planet. Having more energy for our family, kids, and relationship. More energy to put into our business, so we can have a bigger impact and make more income. Having the means and opportunity to see your grandkids grow up; and have plenty of time and energy to play with them.

We start to look at the bigger picture, in our health and across our life. Looking at what is important to us. It's the same with your business, you get to the point where you're asking, "what's next?".

When we attain one goal we naturally start to strive for the next one. We always want what we don't have.

Where do you want to take your business now?

How do you want to expand and grow?

What is my bigger vision?

How can I rule the world?

How to Use This Book...

We'll be going through some of the same success habits you've used in business, and applying them to your body. I'll show you how to apply these in the real world, to see your belt buckle going down a few notches, while your shoulders expand to fill out the sleeves of your suit.

This book is for male entrepreneurs who want to look the part and match their success in business. This is for you if you want to look good in a suit; maybe you do some public speaking or sales, or you have customer facing situations where the way you portray yourself is important to your business. Perhaps you want to be seen and look the part as a leader for your employees.

Your goal might be to get your body to the same high standard that you set in other areas of life, such as your business. To help you not only get the body transformation, but to grow your business as a result. There are two great outcomes from reading and applying these concepts; health, and wealth.

It's for men that value self-improvement. Who want to be on a journey of growth, learning, and development. Always pushing the boundaries, but at the same time being grateful for where they're at right now. You probably value family and freedom. You don't want to be a slave to your business, or to come home at the end of the day too exhausted to spend quality time with the family. You want more time and energy to do the things that you love.

We want to better ourselves, to succeed in business, so that we have more freedom. We're willing to put in the work, but we want the freedom to choose how our time and energy is spent.

If this sounds like you, keep reading...

BUILD

This first section of the book is all about doing the work. It's called 'build' because this is the foundation that everything afterwards is built on top of. This is the part of your journey to having a great physique and a body that serves you, which has the most 'hard work'. We'll be introducing some new habits and behaviours into your daily life that are going to take you to where you want to be.

There will be a period of adjustment, but once you've got used to it, living a healthy lifestyle becomes much easier. We're starting with the first domino for guys in their 30's and 40's, that will set off a cascade effect which makes everything coming afterwards much easier. I like to make things as efficient as possible for my clients, so you can get results with the least amount of time and effort.

That first domino is your testosterone levels.

2 TESTOSTERONE

Get the Testosterone of a 20-Year-Old…

Testosterone is the male hormone for performance. It is what differentiates men from women and gives us many of the masculine characteristics we want and need to succeed in life as an entrepreneur, a father, and a man.

Testosterone is what gives us drive, confidence, and energy as men. It's the basis of our strength, vitality, and passion for building a greater life. Without it, we become a shell of our true potential.

As we get older testosterone levels tend to decrease, which affects our performance in several ways. It affects our drive and aggression as men, which can have an impact on our performance in business. Perhaps we're not turning up with the same 'do whatever it takes' attitude that got us ahead in the first place. It can have an impact on our performance in the gym, with exercise and weight loss. It can have an impact on sexual performance and lower our sex drive as well. Creating knock on effects in our relationships if you're constantly lethargic or struggling to get excited in the bedroom.

Not only does low testosterone reduce our drive, it can also raise anxiety, lower confidence, and decrease energy. If you're lethargic at work, struggling to get through the day without a caffeine drip and sweet 'pick me up' foods every couple of hours, low testosterone might be the problem.

In your twenties your testosterone as a man tends to be at a peak. It's usually after the age of 30 that our natural testosterone levels start to decrease in a significant way. There are ways of slowing that process down and there are ways of maintaining your testosterone levels through the right exercise, proper nutrition, good sleep, and keeping your stress levels down. This is exactly how you create that 'first domino' effect that allows a small tweak here to make a large impact on everything downstream in your health and wellness.

If you're overweight, there is a good chance it is negatively impacting your testosterone levels. Whereas if you stay fit, you can almost entirely avoid the year on year decline in testosterone and all the accompanying negative effects that men tend to see as they pass 30 and beyond.

Testosterone is the first section of this book because it is what I call the first domino. If we can push that domino over, it will create a cascade and all the other dominoes will fall into place. Other things we are going to be looking at in this book will become easier when we have optimised our testosterone levels.

If your testosterone levels are at an optimal level, that's going to have an impact on your performance in the gym. If you can perform better in the gym you're going to have a better body. If you have a better body, you're going to not only look better; you look more presentable and powerful at work, and of course you're going to be healthier as well.

You're going to have more energy, and more drive, if your testosterone is optimised. That's going to transcend into your business. That drive is going to give you more focus, more mojo to be productive at work. If you can be more productive than your competition, because you're properly managing your health and have tons more energy; you're going to blow away your competitors. You're going to make more money and dominate your market. Just by increasing your testosterone level you can see significant changes in your business. Imagine having the energy and drive you had when you started, with the wisdom and experience you have now.

Obviously, this is going to have an impact on your life outside business as well. You're going to have more energy, and more time to spend with your kids. Be more excited to play with them, kick a football around, wrestle, and be the active and involved father that kids love. You're going to have more energy for your wife, be more of a strong, masculine figure and you're going to have better sex. Better sexual performance keeps everyone happy. By optimising your testosterone levels you're going to have more energy to show up and be the best husband and father that you can be. This is where the benefits go far beyond just your own gain, and impact the people closest to you, your loved ones.

If your testosterone levels aren't in the optimal range you're not going to be able to maintain the level of health and optimization you'd ideally want.

You're going to be more stressed and not as well prepared to deal with it. Stress is the biggest killer out there. It leads to problems like heart attacks, strokes, and so much more. Anything to help manage stress is going to be a huge positive in your health and wellness. Stress hormones and testosterone are made from the same pre-cursor materials in the body, so they essentially oppose each other. If you're chronically stressed, the chances are it's lowering your testosterone.

Testosterone is important for the immune system. If you're getting sick, you're not able to exercise, you're not able to produce and perform in your business at the highest level. It's that domino effect. It all works the other way around too. Testosterone can be a negative spiral, or a positive one, depending on a few factors that are generally within your control, which we're going to look at in the coming pages.

A negative spiral of lowering testosterone, increasing sickness, lower energy and lethargy can eventually lead to depression and even early mortality in the worst, most extreme cases, due to lifestyle diseases such as cancer and heart disease.

The way I see it, we're all seeking happiness, we're all looking to live the best life possible. For an entrepreneur your business is important and if you're not performing at the highest level, that can have a psychological impact. As men, as business owners, we're very competitive and when we feel that we're losing that competitive edge, that can have a negative impact on our psychological health.

When that translates into other areas of our life, everything suffers. The time we spend with our kids suffers, quality time spent with our family, the quality of the relationships with your wife, it all starts to suffer when you're being held back from performing at your peak potential and you start bringing your work and a bad mood home with you.

On a physical level because you don't like what you see in the mirror, it affects your confidence. You're not congruent with who you want to be. You want to be a successful guy. Perhaps your success warrants that you should be driving around in a Lamborghini, but your body is more like a Ford Fiesta. There's a level of incongruency there. If you're not carrying a body you're proud of and presenting yourself to the world in a way that you want your business to be represented, there's an incongruence that could be costing you.

What does low testosterone look like?

There are a lot of symptoms that might be showing up to indicate that your testosterone is lower than would be optimal.

One of the indicators is high body fat levels and a good way to check that is to reach down; if you can grab a fistful of belly fat, the chances are your testosterone levels are not going to be anywhere near where you want them to be.

Another simple indicator is to ask if you are pitching a tent in the morning? It's natural for men to have an erection first thing in the morning when they wake up. Not necessarily every morning, but some mornings you should be having an erection. After a good night's sleep, testosterone levels are at their peak first thing when you wake up. That's also a pointer that you do need to get a good night's sleep as well. A lack of sleep will push your hormonal rhythm out of line, and can cause a drop in testosterone levels, and an increase of stress hormones.

The best way to know for certain if you have low testosterone or not is to get a testosterone test done. These are pretty easy. The simplest way of doing it is a saliva test where you just spit into a test tube and the test tube gets sent off to a laboratory to be tested. You get back the results within a week.

This is a proper medical test and will give you the most accurate results. I strongly suggest that every guy gets a testosterone test done to see where they are at. Even if you don't have any symptoms of low testosterone. A baseline testosterone reading will allow you to compare against something in the future. While clinically low testosterone should be treated medically, you should be aiming to get your natural level as high as possible. Being in the normal range is 'ok' but I'd rather see you aiming for the top of the range.

To find out more about getting a testosterone test, and what to do with the results go to www.TheMuscleAndHustleMethod.com/testosterone

Is testosterone really that important?

Absolutely it is. As we said, it's the first domino and if you want to succeed in your body, and beyond, you need to optimize your testosterone. When you do, it will be like taking the handbrake off on your body transformation journey. Finally, you surge forwards, instead of burning through a tank of gas just to creep forwards a few meters.

It's easy to overlook something that we may not be acutely aware of, but it really is that important if you want everything else to fall in to place. Like having the health, the body, the sex drive of a 20-something. If you want to have that drive, that focus in your business that's going to help you blow away the competition, optimising your testosterone is very important and is the logical place to begin.

If you think your testosterone levels are OK, or you don't want to get it tested, that's cool. That's your choice to make. If you do feel that you're suffering from some of the symptoms we talked about; you're not getting an erection in the mornings, if your body fat levels are too high; in my opinion, you should get a test. If those things are not an issue for you, then that's awesome. You probably don't need to worry. Like I said, a baseline reading would still benefit you for the future, regardless of whether you have symptoms now. Practice preventative health care, instead of reactionary 'sick care'.

Even if your levels are good now, if you were able to further optimise your health and performance, to prevent getting sick in the near future, to have more energy, drive, confidence, and to burn fat more easily and build muscle; wouldn't that be worth it?

I want to raise my testosterone. What do I do?

The best way to raise your testosterone levels is to make some simple lifestyle changes. For many guys who do not have clinically low testosterone, or any underlying hormonal problem, it can be done relatively easily. You can raise your testosterone with completely natural methods by changing small lifestyle habits. You don't need any medication, you don't need any drugs, you don't need any steroids to naturally raise your testosterone levels. Simply make some small, simple lifestyle changes and you can reinvigorate your life by raising testosterone back to the levels you had in your younger years. Let's look at some simple tips to help raise your testosterone.

The first place to look when raising your testosterone is to reduce your stress. How do you know if you're too stressed? When you're working all the hour's God sends, you feel like your head's about to explode, you're snappy with your kids, you don't have time to do things you want to do, time for yourself, or the family. When you snap at the smallest things, and all you want to do when you get home is sleep. When there's a black cloud following you around, and it feels like no matter what you do, there's always something else to do around the corner. That's a pretty sure bet that you're too stressed.

You might not even feel stressed. Perhaps you've been pushing so hard for so long, that this intense level of stress just feels normal. If you go on holiday or take a week off over Christmas and suddenly sleep better and feel the weight of the world has been lifted off your chest; you're probably too stressed. To be honest, I could make a sure bet that you would benefit from lower stress levels regardless. Everyone is too stressed nowadays.

The best way to begin reducing stress is with exercise. I recommend lifting weights as a really good way of relieving stress. It releases a lot of tension and channels a lot of aggression. Lifting weights will make you feel strong and confident, which is itself a stress reliever. Getting your heart rate up, blood pumping and being fully present in the moment while you exercise help to wash away the stresses of the day.

Beyond exercise, eating foods that are going to give you more energy is going to help you feel better about yourself. The food you eat is linked with the way your body feels and to your mood. It's important to eat a good, healthy, well-balanced diet. It doesn't necessarily mean you have to spend a lot of time cooking. You can pick up a lot of good, healthy, nutritious food on the go. We'll cover exactly what to eat, as well as how to exercise in the coming chapters.

Finally, aim for six to eight hours of good sleep each night. Try to get to bed and wake up at the same times each day, to keep a nice rhythm. Make your room pitch black and spend at least half an hour winding down before you go to sleep. Reduce screen time late at night to get a more restful night's sleep, reduce stress, and wake up feeling energised.

Those are the three things you can easily add into your life right away, to lower your stress and increase your testosterone levels. There's other things you can do, but these three are the simplest, easiest, and the most all around beneficial lifestyle changes to begin with.

Losing weight is going to have a hugely positive impact on your testosterone levels. The more body fat you carry the more you tend to produce the female sex hormone, estrogen. The higher your estrogen is, the lower your testosterone will be. Being overweight leads to your body turning testosterone into estrogen, which makes you store more fat, as well as increasing risk for multiple lifestyle diseases. You want to avoid that negative spiral by losing weight, which will lower estrogen and raise testosterone.

The leaner, more muscular we can keep ourselves, the more testosterone we will produce. Remember that pinch test we did earlier on? If you can grab a handful of belly fat or more, you could benefit from losing some weight. That's going to boost your testosterone, which then makes it easier to build muscle and lose further weight. Having more muscle mass means your body burns more calories, just to sustain itself. Therefore, adding muscle to your body will also help to reduce your body fat levels. When you get your hormones working for you, they create positive feedback cycles that make weight loss and building a physique exponentially easier.

Aside from being overweight, there are other signals that might indicate you're producing too much estrogen. Your mood for one. You could be feeling emotional, distracted, or just struggle to focus. Maybe you simply don't have the aggression or drive that you used to. If you're overweight, you know that you're going to benefit from losing it.

The best way to lose weight is to start working on yourself. Work on your body and begin exercising. The most effective way to do that would be with weight lifting, which we will explore deeper in the coming chapters. You don't have to spend hours every day in the gym. You can get effective workouts, and great results through as little as three 20 to 30-minute workouts per week. I like to focus my clients on efficiency, rather than trying to make them do more. You're already busy, so we need to find a solution that gets you're the maximum results with the least disruption to your schedule.

Of course, you're not just trying to lose body fat. You want to build muscle as well. Obviously, the best way to do that is through strength training. Again, you only need as little as three 20 to 30-minute workouts per week focusing on compound movements to get stronger and add muscle to your frame. Compound movements are exercises that require the use of more than one muscle group at a time. Things like squats, pushups, and pull ups. When you train with compound movements, you're working multiple muscles at the same time, so you can get the job done in half the time. Train efficiently, rather than spending more time in the gym. You'll discover the specifics of exactly what to do in the chapters about exercise later in the book.

You might have heard that testosterone naturally decreases as you age, beginning around age 30 and accelerating at 40. It does go down naturally as we get older, but you can minimize and dramatically slow that process down by following some of the principles in this book. Just because it normally declines doesn't mean you should roll over and let it happen. Optimising your lifestyle will greatly increase your testosterone levels and essentially allow you to stay younger for longer.

You don't have to helplessly watch your testosterone levels go down as you get older, and see your drive, strength and vitality go with it. You can do something about it. You can do it naturally with the simple lifestyle changes we are discussing here.

You might have read some statistics that say testosterone declines by 1 or 2% every year after the age of 30. That is the case if you don't do anything about it. If you do something about it, that won't be the case for you. Simply make the lifestyle changes discussed in this book and you can reduce and even reverse much of the age-related decline of testosterone levels.

Perhaps it seems like the easy answer is to just take steroids. To shortcut doing any work and just get to the end by artificial means. That is perhaps partly true, but obviously steroids can have some not-so-positive side effects. Even if you were to take steroids, that doesn't necessarily mean you're going to get results. Steroids won't have the effect you're looking for without the correct exercise and correct nutrition in place anyway. I guess one way I could describe it is a well-known bodybuilder from the 60s, Tom Platz described it as, "You wouldn't wax a dirty car".

You must have everything else in place and be following the correct protocols. The exercise, the nutrition, and the rest. The lifestyle must be in place for steroids, or any supplement, to have any kind of positive effect on your body. Otherwise you're risking your health in hopes of a quick-fix that is never going to work. Focus on the basics; food, exercise, and sleep.

Of course, there is a difference between taking steroids, like a bodybuilder might, and hormone replace therapy (HRT) recommended by a doctor. Always take the advice of your doctor if that is what he or she recommends. Just bear in mind, there's many things you can do naturally before the use of steroids. Even before going on HRT, making lifestyle changes might be enough. It might not fix the problem, but even if it doesn't, your general health and wellbeing will be so much better you will get exponentially more benefits if you do need to go on HRT.

A doctor's job is generally to prescribe something, because that's the easiest and quickest thing to do. The issue is that it doesn't address the real problem. Doctors usually want to prescribe a pill to relieve the pain, without addressing where the pain is coming from. Of course, this is just how the system is set up. Doctors on an individual level are great people who dedicate their lives to helping others, but the system is set up in such a way where they only see each person for 5-10 minutes and are very limited in what they can do to help. Not to mention, even after telling people to change their lifestyle, most people are not committed enough to do it, and demand a 'quick fix' anyway. To take control of your body, and life, question what is causing a problem with your testosterone? It could be a serious illness, but statistically it is more likely poor lifestyle choices, bad diet, lack of exercise, and excess stress.

You might find that if you get a test, your doctor says your results are within the normal range, but you still have some of the symptoms. Your testosterone levels could be 'ok' and you still might have the symptoms. We know that exercise, nutrition, sleep, and a healthy lifestyle will boost your levels even more. Living a healthier lifestyle has no downside, and lots of upside. No matter where you are regarding your testosterone - or any other part of your health – a healthier lifestyle is always a net positive. Indeed, there is no downside to being healthier. Especially when you make it as efficient as possible, so as not to distract from other important parts of your life.

Living a healthy lifestyle is the best way to reduce body fat, build muscle, increase your performance, energy, and drive. There is no loss from living a healthier lifestyle, even if it didn't boost your testosterone levels, you'd still get massive benefit from it in every part of your day to day life.

I'm not recommending the use of steroids in any way in this chapter, but rather placing your focus on what you can do naturally to increase your testosterone levels. Testosterone is extremely important, but it is also very much within your control to change, without resorting to steroids.

If you decide for whatever reason that you don't want to get tested, that is fine. You don't have to get tested. As I said, there are some indicators that your testosterone levels might be low based on how much body fat you're carrying, your sex drive, whether you're having erections in the morning. These are good indicators. Be aware of these things and account for them. If you notice you're having problems in these areas, I would recommend you get a test to ensure you have all the data at hand to make the best decisions for your long-term health.

To start boosting your testosterone you just need to take action, take that first step. You either get yourself in the gym, or if you don't have time for that, do something at home. Get yourself out for a 10 to 15-minute walk. The hardest thing to do is start, so that's the most important thing to do. To begin with just do the easiest thing that's going to get you started.

Go to www.TheMuscleAndHustleMethod.com/testosterone to find out more in-depth information about testosterone testing.

Optimised Testosterone Checklist

- ✓ Can you grab less than a fistful of belly fat?
- ✓ Do you wake up with an erection more than 3 times per week?
- ✓ Are you not over your ideal weight?
- ✓ Is your energy and mood consistently stable?

Testosterone in the Real World

Let me illustrate some of the benefits you can get by simply making the correct lifestyle choices. I recently had my client Iain take a testosterone test. He's 52 and the results came back a week later at 109.8. That's the equivalent of a man half his age, which is very impressive, but it wasn't always like that.

Iain runs his own building business. As you can imagine, he followed a typical builders lifestyle. Early starts, a daily fry up in the local greasy spoon cafe, work all day, then down the pub with the lads for a few pints after work. When we started working together, Iain was heavily overweight at 96kg and had a big beer belly, as you can imagine after years living this kind of lifestyle. While working together Iain has made some small healthy changes to his diet and incorporated some short effective workouts that have resulted in him dropping 16kg (35lbs), losing the belly, getting more done at work, and having the testosterone levels of a 20-something again.

Plus, he still has a few pints and the odd fry up from time to time. He didn't have to totally change his life or give up things he likes to achieve this. Iain's returned to running and recently ran a 10k race in just over an hour. Something he used to do a lot in his 20's. He also attends a weekly boxing class, where he has made some friends that support and motivate him. I can't emphasise the importance of environment and who you hang around with enough. If you work in an environment where everybody bitches and complains, its likely you will bitch and complain. If all your mates like going to the pub to get hammered every night, you're probably going to do the same. Hang around with fit and healthy people, it's likely you will be fit and healthy. That's just the way it is. They say you are the sum of the 5 people you spend the most time with, so choose your friends wisely. Here's what Iain said about what motivated him to make a change in his life.

"It started when I noticed it was getting difficult to put my shoes on in the morning without getting out of breath and my trousers in the wardrobe did not fit any more. For the last couple of years, I've known I had to stop smoking, I knew it was causing me harm, but I was also aware that most people put on weight after stopping. I couldn't afford to gain any more weight, indeed I needed to lose some, so I decided that I should link the two ideas and go for a complete change of lifestyle.

Funnily I found that going to the gym and getting fitter only increased my resolve to stop smoking and rather than making the process more difficult, my new-found fitness routine became an aid to help me stop smoking. 7 or 8 months into the process when I started going to classes I found the social aspect also helped to provide motivation for those early mornings.

To sum up, I would say that my decision came from a gradual realisation that I had to reverse the effects my lifestyle was having on my weight and overall health. Going to the gym and working with Ed provided accountability and a structure to the process. I'm not sure that I had any specific fears, more a general awareness that my lifestyle was not sustainable, and I would find it increasingly difficult to do the things I wanted to do if I continued on this path. I was aware that as I got older time was slipping away and if I didn't take action soon, it was only going to get more difficult".

After a year of making lifestyle changes, working out and making simple switches to his nutrition Iain is healthier than he has been for years, has bucket loads of energy, and a new lease on life. Plus, the testosterone that makes many guys in their 20's envious.

Testosterone Conclusions

Testosterone is the male sex hormone. For women, its estrogen. We all have both hormones in our body, but for us guys the ratio of testosterone is far greater than estrogen, and vice versa for women. Well it should be anyway, if you're healthy.

Testosterone really is the big domino. It's what makes a man a man! Imagine being told by your GP that you have the testosterone levels of a 3-year-old girl. You're in bed with your missus and you can't get it up. What do you think's going through her head? She's thinking you're not attracted to her anymore. You're thinking I can't satisfy my wife and it's only a matter of time before she cheats on me with a younger man who does have the energy to give her what she needs. As you can see, low testosterone levels can have a huge impact on you psychologically, as well as physically. It can really affect your state of mind in negative ways.

I remember when I had man boobs, and how that affected me. Man boobs are often linked to a hormonal imbalance, specifically high estrogen levels. I hated the way my body looked and never wanted to take my t-shirt off on the beach. In fact, I would wear a t-shirt over my t-shirt and do anything I could to hide my man boobs. I was self-conscious about getting undressed in front of women. Looking back now, I think this had an impact on me even talking to women. I mean, I've always been a shy, introverted guy anyway, so chatting to women has never been my strong point but having low self-confidence certainly didn't help matters as I tended to shy away from even trying, because I didn't think I was good enough. I don't want you to find yourself in a similar situation. If you want to find out more about how testosterone impacts your health, or how to get your testosterone tested, go to www.TheMuscleAndHustleMethod.com/testosterone.

3 NUTRITION

In the previous section we have touched on the importance of nutrition in terms of how it impacts your testosterone levels. Of course, the impact that nutrition has on your health and body goes far beyond that. What you eat is the fuel you are feeding your body and brain to function throughout the day. Are you feeding it nutritious, energising foods or things that make you sluggish and heavy?

Nutrition is the greatest input that you have direct control over when it comes to your weight and physical shape. You are always in control of what you eat, and therefore always have the power to gain or lose weight by modifying your intake. Nutrition can be a complicated topic and we're just going to distil the information down into the simple, actionable big levers you need to know to see the results you're looking for. In this chapter you're going to discover how to lose the belly, while still eating foods you enjoy. Let's get started.

Eat What You Want.

Wish you could simplify nutrition? It's so complicated that many people never see the results they're looking for, because they simply don't know where to start. Let me break down the things you need to know. Like I said in the introduction of this book, I've tried just about every diet out there, and I know from experience that most of them do not work. Why? Nutrition is one of those topics that has a lot of conflicting information out there. So many diets that are given a fancy name, but they all mean one thing and that is simply to eat less. Eat less calories and you will lose weight.

There's better ways of doing that, in a way that's not restrictive to yourself, or is easier to follow. You can still eat all the foods that you want to eat, that you enjoy, if you don't overdo it. You can eat them in a way that's part of a plan which is still reducing your overall calories. You might need to eat less of them, but you don't have to give them up entirely. Losing weight is not about the specific food you're eating, or cutting out different food groups, or specific nutrients. The most important thing is how much you're eating and your portion sizes. Let me repeat: It's not which foods you're eating, it's how much you're eating.

Nutrition is important. It's your fuel. If you drive a nice car you wouldn't put the wrong fuel in it. You'd not only put the correct fuel in, you'd probably put premium fuel in there for optimized performance. It's just the same with your body. You are what you eat. If you're going to eat junk all the time, then that's how you're going to look and feel. If you eat good, nutritious, healthy food then you're going to look good, you're going to feel good, you're going to have a better mood, you're going to have more optimized performance and better drive.

Eating nutritious food to fuel your body doesn't mean you can't still enjoy a little bit of 'junk food' here and there. It's all about the balance. Eating everything in moderation is a much more sustainable approach and is a much healthier lifestyle than an overly strict plan that eliminates various foods or groups of foods. It will allow you to get great results, but also sustain and keep those results for the rest of your life. Trying to cut foods or entire food groups out of your diet isn't a sustainable way to live, and makes you hate what you're doing. You'll not follow it forever and always end up going back the other direction with a binge. What's the point of torturing yourself with a routine you hate for a few weeks, only to regress back to where you started anyway?

Having just said you can eat some 'junk food' every now and then, that is not encouragement to base your diet on it. When you eat crappy food, and more importantly when you eat too much of it, you're going to feel sluggish. When you eat junk all you want to do is curl up in a ball on the sofa and sleep or reach for a coffee because your energy levels have crashed. Think what happens mid-morning after you eat a croissant and sugary coffee for breakfast. Whereas if you eat something more nutritious you're going to feel energized. You're going to feel awake and alive, ready and raring to go for the day ahead. After eating a good meal you're going to feel recharged, which is precisely how you should feel after fueling yourself with the nutrients your body needs.

When you get back to work after a healthy lunch you're going to be much more productive than if you eat junk and want to fall sleep, are sluggish and don't want to even look at a computer screen. All you're going to want to do is have a nap if you're putting the wrong fuel in your body. Putting aside weight loss and health; which do you think is more productive for your business? Time is money. If you fall asleep for an hour, dependent on your hourly rate how much is that going to cost you? If you're someone who charges £500, or £1,000 an hour, how much is it costing you in lost productivity and income to fall asleep for that hour? Imagine what you could get done if you fueled yourself properly every day.

Let me tell you about a client of mine, Gavin. Gavin is an example of a successful weight loss story without going on a diet and giving up all his favourite foods, or the odd beer. Gavin lost 28lbs in 12 weeks while working with me, while still enjoying food and drinks like he always has.

When Gavin initially approached me, he was heavily overweight through a lifestyle of inactivity, rich food and too much beer. He wasn't comfortable in his own skin or in the clothes he wore. It was severely affecting his self-confidence. He wasn't living the life he wanted to.

This held him back from getting in the gym and doing something about his weight. He was too worried about what others thought of him, because he didn't have a clue what he was doing. He felt like the gym was full of fit and healthy people and he didn't fit in there. The truth is, people are not looking at you or judging you, the vast majority of the time. Even on a very rare occasion, if they are, so what? That's more of a reflection on them than it is on you. You shouldn't let others affect or determine the outcome you want to achieve. We all had to start somewhere on our journey. It was day 1 in the gym for everyone, once upon a time.

We had to take baby steps to help Gav overcome this. Not by giving him a complicated program to follow. The most important step was that he walked through the gym door. This was a big achievement at the beginning. It didn't matter what workout he did. His first workouts consisted of walking for 10 minutes on the treadmill. It was all about getting him into the gym and building some consistency into his routine.

Once he became confident going to the gym, we started to give him some simple but effective exercises to do. It's important to start at the appropriate level. A complicated workout program that is supposed to be 'more effective' isn't going to work if it's intimidating and you never actually walk through the gym doors to do it.

Anyway, back to Gavin's 'no diet' diet. Gavin has always been a social person. He likes his food and loves cooking for friends and enjoying a few beers. We had to work with this, rather than against it. We didn't want to take away or restrict him from doing the things he loves. One of the biggest mistakes people make when trying to lose weight, is they restrict themselves too much with a 'diet' and cutting out things they enjoy like their favourite foods and booze. Now they're doing something they hate and can't wait to stop. Does that sound sustainable to you?

Willpower and discipline will only carry you so far. With Gavin we knew that we had to make some changes but didn't want to take away all the things he enjoys doing, like cooking and having a drink. He had tried this in the past. He gave up drinking, went on a diet, and lost a load of weight. Of course, he ended up putting it all and even more back on, as soon as he went 'back to normal'.

This time round, I never asked him to give up beer, but he was able to commit to reducing it a little bit. I didn't ask him to change what he cooked or what he was eating, but he was able to commit to reducing his portion sizes slightly and eating less junk between meals. Add to that the fact that he was going to the gym, which Gavin started to enjoy once he got into it and was happy going 4-5 times a week.

These small and manageable changes quickly added up. Gavin was able to drop 28lbs in the 12 weeks we were working together. To start wearing his best clothes again and feel more confident, all without any drastic changes or restrictions to his life.

By not restricting yourself in any way, it's more likely this will become a habit and a sustainable part of your life. I recently checked in with Gav and he continues to regularly attend the gym and has lost further weight. Building simple changes into your lifestyle, instead of trying to change everything and become a perfect robotic 'fitness guy' works. Not only does it work, but it's infinitely more enjoyable than trying to cut out all the things you like doing. Wouldn't you like to lose weight, get fitter and healthier; with just some simple changes that are easy to follow and don't make you feel miserable about doing it?

What does a healthy diet or good nutrition look like?

A healthy diet is something that's going to fuel your goals. If you want to present to the world a strong, masculine figure, you need to eat in such a way as to create that. This requires good food with high-protein, a moderate amount of carbs, and a moderate amount of fats in your diet.

For protein that will be high quality lean meats; chicken, turkey, steak, fish, and eggs. Plenty of green vegetables or salads to go with it for fiber and micronutrients. For energy a moderate amount of carbohydrates from natural, clean foods such as potatoes, rice, pasta, and bread in moderate amounts.

Yes, you can eat bread and pasta if you want (if you don't have a wheat intolerance). Bread and pasta doesn't make us fat. Eating too much of it makes us fat. Like eating too much of anything will make you fat.

Fats should come from natural sources like olive oil, oily fish, coconut oil, nuts, avocado, and those that are naturally contained in meat, fish, and eggs.

For each meal simply choose a good quality protein source as the base of the meal. Choose a good quality carbohydrate for energy as required. Carbs provide energy, but they are not essential all the time. I tend to have them at my most active times of day, for example the meal before or after a workout. Then a small amount of fats keeps you feeling full as well to keep your hormones and brain functioning at an optimal level with the nutrients they need.

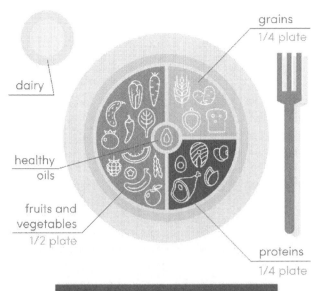

grains
1/4 plate

dairy

healthy
oils

fruits and
vegetables
1/2 plate

proteins
1/4 plate

HEALTHY PLATE

This is nutritious, healthy food, but if you're eating too much of it, you've still got the same problem. You're still going to be overweight, you're still going to be fat if you overeat 'healthy food'. Calories count, and even in healthy, nutritious food; too much is too much. Although healthier food tends to be lower in calories, it will still make you fat if you overeat it. As I said it's not the food you're eating, it's the amount of food you're eating. You could still be fat eating chicken, broccoli, and rice, if you eat too much of it.

You might be 'eating healthy' but it's calories that count at the end of the day. If you're still consuming too many calories then you're going to be overweight, you're going to be out of shape, and you're going to be lethargic because of it.

You don't need to eat the chicken and broccoli out of Tupperware deal. It doesn't have to be bland and boring. Preparing meals is fine if that's what you want to do, but you could just as easily go to your local supermarket, pick up a pre-cooked protein source, grab some fruit or something on the go and eat that. Or you could pick up food from a takeout place that serves healthy meals in just a couple of minutes or less. Fast food doesn't have to be bad for you, or packed full of calories.

If you need to eat between meals you can grab a high protein snack such as beef jerky, a protein bar, Greek yoghurt, or some nuts. If you need an energy boost, a piece of fruit usually does the trick, or you could get some rice or oat cakes and spread a little peanut butter and a drizzle of honey on top. This is a nice little snack that I enjoy, and it keeps me from reaching for the biscuits. These are ideal snacks that you could just grab and go or can keep handy in the office or in your bag if you're travelling. They don't require any cooking or warming up, and other than the Greek yoghurt and fruit, they don't even need to be kept chilled.

I tend to eat a little bit more in the evenings for dinner. Personally, I prefer to keep my eating during the day quite light. I just snack in the way I described above and have a bigger dinner like many people enjoy. I usually workout in the evening, so I need the extra fuel. This keeps my metabolism revved up, so I'm in an optimum fat-burning state, my muscles and brain fueled for the day.

Nutrition doesn't have to be complicated, or dogmatic. Just account for your overall calories, and do what works for your schedule, while keeping you fueled and feeling good throughout the day. What I'm saying might well be simpler and easier than you would have thought. The truth is it is simple and easy to eat right. People giving you overly complicated plans are just trying to bamboozle you with complexity into thinking you *need* to buy their products to understand what to do. You don't. You just need to understand a few basic principles, and then apply a little conscious thought to what you're doing. The only plan that works, is your own one. The one that you can follow and enjoy over the long term.

I'm just like you. I'm a busy guy. I don't have the time to spend hours in the kitchen cooking my meals. Just because I opt for convenience doesn't mean eating rubbish. Fast food doesn't have to mean you go and get a pizza, burger, or something like that. Fast food can be healthy as well. It's quick and convenient. Speed and convenience is the key for me. I always look for meals that I can grab and go. I don't want to have to cook, I don't want to have to clean up and do the dishes afterwards. I just want something I can quickly open and put together a very simple, quick, and easy meal that's going to give me the protein I need to build and repair my muscles and give me the energy I need to get through the day. Not only to get through the day, but to give me enough energy to work out hard, produce in my business, and spend quality time with my family and kids.

The food you eat is your fuel. Many people simply eat for the sake of eating. Whereas if you see your food as fuel and eat according to your energy demands, you're less likely to store excess food as body fat. For example, if you have some carbs, they will provide energy. But if you're sitting at a desk all day, you might not necessarily need that energy. If you're on the go, you're on your feet all day then your demand for more food and more carbohydrates would be greater.

If you're about to go to the gym, you're going to require more energy for that and should adjust your food accordingly. Have slightly more carbohydrates around those times. The mistake a lot of people tend to make, they go for high carb, high fat, low protein foods, because they tend to be the easiest most convenient foods to get hold of when you're on the go. Opting for something high protein and healthy can be just as easy and convenient. It simply requires a tiny bit more thought and awareness.

Another common mistake is that most people usually have their biggest meal in the evening when they've finished work and they're just kicking back, relaxing. While during the day they haven't fueled themselves as much as needed to perform their daily tasks. If you're winding down for the day, you don't need that amount of food in the evening. Of course, if you haven't fueled yourself throughout the day you're probably getting home starving hungry and looking forward to a nice big feast.

If you haven't had anything for breakfast and gone all day without eating, it's no surprise that you're going to want to eat a big meal. It's important to get some regular meals and snacks in throughout the day so your energy is consistent, and your body always has the fuel it needs. Then you can enjoy a nice meal in the evening with the family, but you don't feel the need to overeat.

Here's an example of a 'grab and go' diet for someone who works out in the evening.

- ✓ Breakfast 8am - Egg sandwich/breakfast bap and a coffee from your chosen coffee shop.

- ✓ Snack 11am - Handful of cashew nuts

- ✓ Lunch 1pm – Cooked, sliced chicken breast and a handful of ready washed spinach leaves from the supermarket.

- ✓ Snack 4pm - 2 rice cakes with peanut butter.

✓ WORKOUT 6pm

✓ Dinner 8pm - Salmon fillet, baked potato and broccoli.

Understanding What You're Eating

The best way to figure out what you're eating, and what will be the correct amount for you, is by tracking your food intake. You can easily do this using the My Fitness Pal app on your smart phone. You can track your calories using the app, and it will track your activity levels too, to work out the level of intake you need. It's really easy to do. It doesn't mean you have to log your food all the time. You could just do it for a day or two, to get an idea of how much you're consuming.

The more informed you are, the more data you have to inform your decisions, the better off you will be. I strongly recommend everyone tracks their food at least for a few days, just to start gaining an understanding of how much you're eating, and the energy density of different kinds of foods.

If you don't have time for tracking what you eat all the time, I tell my clients to use their hand as a guide. Use the palm of your hand to determine your portion sizes. Aim to eat an amount of protein equivalent to the size of your palm, and the same amount of carbohydrates.

Most importantly when you're tracking your food is to look at overall calories to begin with. How do you know if you're having too many calories? You can put into My Fitness Pal your information such as age, height, weight, and activity levels and it will give you an estimate of how many calories you typically need throughout the day.

Obviously if you're going in excess of that number, you know you're eating too much. Meanwhile, if you're way under that number you may need to eat a little bit more. Nutrition is not complicated, simply eat approximately the right number of calories, consistently, and you will see the outcomes you're looking for.

A simple way to keep tabs on progress if your goal is weight loss is to weigh yourself. If you're not losing any weight, you know that you need to reduce your portions or total calories a little bit. It really is not more complicated than that. If you're trying to lose weight, and the scales are not moving down, you're eating too much. If they're going down, keep doing what you're doing.

If you're not seeing the progress you want, either reduce your portions a little bit or exercise a bit more to burn a few extra calories. The simple formula for weight loss is to be in a calorie deficit. That can be achieved in two ways. Either to eat a little bit less or move a bit more. If the needle on the scales is not moving, you need to adjust one of those two variables until it does. This is totally within your control and hopefully understanding this is demystifying 'dieting' for you. Simply eat more or less as needed, depending on your calorie needs, and the goal you're trying to achieve. Your weight will tell you if you're going in the right direction or not.

To set up and use My Fitness Pal go to www.myfitnesspal.com or download the app on your smart phone. Set up your account.

Next is to input your goals. The app will ask you to enter your current weight, and your desired goal weight, along with some other information like your sex, height, age, and activity levels. It will use this information to work out your calorie requirements for your desired goal.

You're now good to go and you can start tracking your foods. My Fitness Pal has a huge database of foods from all over the world, including all the major brands and restaurants. Even many of the smaller brands. You'll be surprised how effective it is. You can simply scan the barcode of your grab and go foods using your phones camera, add it to your food diary or type in the search bar to find your food if it doesn't have a bar code to scan.

It's quite good fun as well as an eye opener, understanding the nutrient density of the foods you're eating. You might be surprised at how many calories are in some of the foods you typically eat.

After making sure we're consuming the right number of calories we look at our macros, or macronutrients. Macros are protein, carbohydrates, and fats. Your overall calories are made up of these three macronutrients. What's most important for body composition is getting the right balance of macronutrients. Calories affect overall weight loss/weight gain most, but when it comes to the shape of your body, macros play an important role.

The balance of macronutrients you need vary from person to person, obviously depending on activity levels and your metabolism. A general rule of thumb for body composition - building muscle and losing fat - is to consume around one gram of protein per pound of body weight, or two pounds per kilogram of bodyweight. After you have your protein intake at the correct level, your remaining calories can come from carbs and fats.

Within the boundaries of your macros you can eat whatever you want. Or to put it another way, you can eat any foods you desire, as long as you are meeting the right macros at the end of the day. If you hit those numbers, you can do that eating whatever food you want. The beauty of tracking your macros is you can eat pretty much what you want, if it fits your macros.

The thing to bear in mind with flexible dieting is; it's one thing to hit those numbers, but you probably don't want to be doing it eating junk food all the time. That wouldn't be in the best interests of health. You could eat crappy food everyday as long as you're hitting those macros. You will lose weight and reach your body composition goals if you do that, but as we said earlier, the quality of the food you're eating has a big impact on your health, your mood, the way you feel, and your energy levels. You could lose weight eating just fast food if you wanted, but your body certainly won't look as good on the inside as it will on the outside. Bare this in mind when you're choosing how to eat. Fitting something into your macro plan isn't license to eat crap and think it isn't going to negatively impact your health. It's important to be healthy on the inside too. The point I'm trying to make is that you don't have to restrict yourself from the foods you like. You can have 'treat' foods, or 'naughty' foods every once in a while. Just don't have them every day. It's all about finding that balance that you enjoy, gives you some freedom, but brings results.

Most people want to focus on improving their body composition and that means you need to focus on protein. Hitting your protein goal is the top priority every day. It's the same as having daily targets within our business. If you're eating out, opt for high-protein food, such as lean meat or fish. Protein should always be your priority. If you go into the supermarket, go to the section where you're going to pick up some protein. Normally people go to the sandwich section at the front of the supermarket, but if you go to the section where you can pick up some pre-cooked meat, you can get things like roast chicken breast, shredded beef, cooked fish, smoked salmon, etc. Even if you want a meat-free option, a good alternative would be Greek yogurt, cottage cheese, or eggs. You can even pick up protein bars and ready-to-drink protein shakes in the supermarket these days.

Not to mention, there's so many meal preparation and food delivery services available online now. I recommend this to a lot of my clients. As a busy entrepreneur, your time should be focused on your business. How good would it be to outsource something like this? No more time spent cooking, cleaning, shopping for food. You can have your food freshly prepared to your exact calorie and macro nutrient requirements and delivered to your door every day. I personally have used a meal prep and delivery service during busier times in my life and its awesome! You have everything you need on your doorstep, so there's no reason you can't eat right, even if you're very busy or too pushed for time to do it yourself.

If tracking is not your thing or you don't have time for it then I would always, as a rule of thumb, choose to eat something high in protein ahead of anything else. Rather than the sandwiches or the cookies and donuts that are always on offer at the front of the supermarket. Find yourself something high in protein and you're half way there when it comes to succeeding on your diet plan.

Even if you don't cook your own meals, using this simple framework you will be much better off than if you just default to eating anything else or if you don't think about it at all and continue to do what you've been doing.

How about carbohydrates?

Carbohydrates and fats are the main sources of energy that your body burns. For carbohydrates I would recommend to just use them accordingly when you need. When you feel that you need an energy boost, or you've worked out hard. If you're sitting at your desk all day you probably don't need many carbs, and that includes not eating too much fruit. You need to be burning energy to earn the need to eat a lot of carbohydrates.

The best time to have carbs is when you first wake up, with your breakfast. Have some protein and carbohydrates for breakfast, which might be some fruit, oats, or bread. Then have the bulk of your other carbohydrates before and after activity such as working out. If you're going to go to the gym in the afternoon then you might want to have some carbs around lunchtime, and perhaps after your workout. If you're going to go to the gym in the evening after work, you might want to have some carbs in the evening. Some people say not to have any carbs after 6:00pm but if you're at your most active after 6:00pm then there's nothing wrong with doing that. The carbohydrates you eat will fuel your workout and recovery as your muscles get stronger. There is no need to follow arbitrary dogma. Simply look at when you most need the energy and consume it around those times. Carbs are not the enemy and there's certainly no need to cut them out of your diet completely.

For fats I recommend you have a moderate amount throughout the day. If your diet is high protein, then chances are you'll be getting a reasonable amount of fats too. You'll be getting some fats from eating meat, fish, and eggs, and from oils you use in cooking (I recommend olive oil or coconut oil). However, if you're having very lean meats all the time like white fish and chicken breast, then you might want to get an additional fat source in there which could come from a handful of nuts, nut butters which goes very nice on oat cakes and rice cakes, salad dressings, olive oil, that kind of thing. Alternatively, you can go for the higher-fat meats, oily fish like mackerel or salmon, steaks, lamb, chicken, and turkey if you leave the skin on. If you have those higher-fat meats, there'll be less of a need for other additional fat sources.

Fats are calorie dense, containing 9 calories per gram, compared to 4 calories per gram in protein and carbohydrates, so you don't want to eat too many fatty foods. They're not 'bad' for your health at all, but it is easy to overeat too many calories. If you're going to eat nuts, have a handful, not a bag full.

You don't need to eliminate carbs or eliminate fat. Carbs don't make you fat. Fats don't make you fat. Consuming too many calories makes you fat, whatever food that might be. You should not be eliminating anything. We need all the macronutrients to function properly, to have energy and optimum health.

It's important to have a moderate amount of fats in the diet. They're important for a number of body processes and are called 'essential fatty acids' for a reason – we need them! The mistake a lot of people tend to make is they have too many carbs, too many fats, and not enough protein; which is why their body composition skews towards having a higher body fat level. They're getting in too much unused energy from an intake of too many carbohydrates and too much fat that's not being used up as fuel. Make protein and vegetables the base of your diet, and consume carbs and fat as needed to boost your energy.

Example Diet Plan

For someone who exercises and requires more energy in the afternoon.

8am - 2 scrambled eggs and smoked salmon on 1 slice of toast

11am - 170g Greek yoghurt with 40g oats and a drizzle of honey.

1pm - EXERCISE

2pm - Whey Protein and peanut butter smoothie with a banana.

4pm 100g cooked chicken breast salad.

7pm 150g steak and green vegetables.

What about drinks? What should I be drinking?

Make sure you drink plenty of water throughout the day. You need to stay hydrated, and water is a basic human need. If you're not drinking enough water you're going to feel sluggish, low energy, and struggle to concentrate. Indeed, often when people are thirsty they use food, especially sugar, as a pick-me-up. Drinking more water can help you lose weight, just by giving you more energy, which naturally cuts down on the sugary snacks.

You've got to bear in mind, calories don't just come from food, they come from drinks as well. If you're having a lot of high calorie drinks; lattes, hot chocolates, if you're drinking soft drinks, even juices contain a lot of calories. The best way to hydrate yourself without taking in an excess of calories would be to just drink water, which doesn't have any calories of course. It hydrates you and has everything you need. Drinking calories is an easy way to take in lots of calories, without feeling full or satisfied like you do with food, so is best kept to a minimum or avoided all together.

What about booze? You can still have an occasional drink. If you do want to have a drink, just remember to take it into consideration in your overall caloric intake, or it is going to put you way over your calorie requirements and lead to you storing unwanted body fat. Alcohol tends to be high in calories, and many people drink a lot once they get started. It's a very easy way to consume too many calories, while receiving no nutritional value. That said, I know people – myself included – like to have a drink. There's the whole social aspect of it, and this is exactly where a sensible approach is best. Restricting yourself and saying you will never drink won't work, because it disrupts your life and you're taking away something you enjoy. Simply be sensible, account for the calories, and find a way to fit them into your overall weekly goal.

Snacking vs Structured Meals?

There is not a right or wrong answer here, it is simply what works for you. For most people I would recommend you snack throughout the day and try to avoid going long hours without eating. Aim to eat a little meal, regularly throughout the day. Eat every three to four hours if possible. You can have some kind of food, it doesn't have to be a big meal, it could be a snack like a handful of nuts, or a protein bar. Just keep yourself feeling satisfied and your energy levels consistent across the day. If you have more free time, then structured meals might work better for you, but the reality is that most of us are short on time.

The best way to ensure you're getting all the food you need is to structure and plan out your day. One of the little habits I have is to block out my meal times. I block out around half an hour per meal. This came from a few years back when I had braces fitted, and it would literally take me 30 minutes to eat something, even a banana. I needed to make sure I set enough time between clients to eat as I was prepping for a fitness competition at the time. So missing meals wasn't an option for me. The meal times have stuck in my diary ever since. I'll have my breakfast in the morning first thing, and I'll block out half an hour mid-morning around 11:30-ish for a snack. Then I'll block out lunch around 1:30- 2:00. Then an afternoon snack around 4:30 just to make sure that I'm getting those meals in and I'm prepared. Otherwise you get caught up in work or doing other tasks. You end up finishing work, you're hungry and you're just going to reach for the quickest and most convenient thing; which is rarely the thing that is going to be the best choice. By blocking out time to eat, you ensure you're doing what you need to do, and it breaks up your day nicely too.

My client Gavin who I mentioned earlier came to me, when he was 18 stone 2lbs. He likes cooking, he likes cooking for friends and family. He's a very social eater and drinker and this was an important part of his lifestyle. We just put him through a 12-week transformation and he lost 24 pounds in just under 12 weeks. What he told me was that he's been a bit more sensible with his diet, he's been a bit more prepared. He's doing his shopping in advance, just so he's properly prepared. What he found is that he hasn't had to give up eating everything he likes, or the social aspects of food and drink that he loves.

What he's done in the past is gone on a diet and he's lost the weight but ended up putting it back on shortly afterwards because the plan he followed has been unsustainable. He's lost it too quickly, by making too many drastic changes to his lifestyle. This time round we've still managed to lose the weight quickly, but he's been cooking for his friends and family, and doing everything that he loves around food. He loves to cook a roast dinner, and he's still been eating that every weekend. He's still been going out, he's a very social person as well and likes to get out regularly. Sometimes he can go out three times a week, which would normally involve drinking a lot of beer. He's still been going out, he's still been having a few beers, but not to the excess that he was doing.

He's brought some balance into his life, where he's been a little bit healthier, made some small changes, but he's not restricting himself from doing the things that he loves doing. He loves cooking for his friends, he loves eating with his friends, he enjoys going out with his friends and having a few drinks. He still enjoys doing all those things, he just brought a little bit of a healthy balance into his life.

He's lost 28 pounds and he feels in a much stronger position to keep the weight off because he's not come to the end of the process and felt like, "I can't wait to have a drink", or "I can't wait to go and eat this or that". He's still eating those things and he's still doing those things. It's just a more sustainable approach that he can enjoy, instead of putting his life on hold to try and lose weight, to just return to doing exactly what he did before as soon as he 'finishes the diet'.

The primary action point for this chapter is to focus on portion sizes. By tracking calories using My Fitness Pal, or if you don't have time for that, just use the palm of your hand as a guide and focus on eating a protein rich meal. Aim to eat one palm of protein at each meal. Try not to restrict yourself or cut out all your favourite foods. Likewise, don't completely change your routine and isolate yourself from social aspects of food and drinking that you enjoy. Simply eat the right number of calories, by being prepared, and snacking throughout the day to keep your energy levels consistent. With this style of eating you can lose weight, increase your energy, and feel great; without having to give up all your favourite foods or totally change your lifestyle.

4 EXERCISE

If you just want to lose weight and are not interested in building muscle or being in better shape, then you can do that with diet alone. Don't get me wrong, exercise certainly helps, but it is a relatively minor part of the equation. Where exercise is important is for transforming how you look, how you feel, and of course your health. To look good, have a strong and commanding presence, you need to build some muscle and strength, to stand up tall and fill out your shoulders.

Health wise, exercise is important for a strong heart and lungs, slowing the ageing process and keeping you looking and feeling younger. It also helps to raise your natural testosterone levels as mentioned in the first section of this book.

There are 2 options for exercise in my recommendations. The first is for someone who is new to exercise, or very short on time; and mostly focused on weight loss. Then there are recommendations for people who want to look better, have more muscle, bigger arms, chest, and shoulders; better posture and a stronger presence. Both are based on efficiency, and designed to get you the most benefit, for the least amount of time and effort. The first principle is consistent; regardless of your goals…

Train Less Than You Think

Do you want to flatten your stomach and fill your shirt sleeves in less than two hours a week?

Contrary to conventional opinion, you can get a good workout done in less than two hours each week, when you do the right things. You could train three times a week, 20 to 40-minute sessions and get fantastic results. You can build muscle that's going to allow you to fill out your shirt in all the right places, while reducing your waist line so that your belt buckle reduces by a couple of notches.

The most important thing is intensity, not quantity, when it comes to exercise. You don't necessarily have to train for hours and hours, or train like an athlete. What you find is that even some of the top athletes don't train for longer than 45 minutes to an hour per day. It's a bit like running your business. The more productive you are, the more work you're going to get done in less time. It's the same with your workouts. Be more productive, train smart, train hard. Not necessarily train longer or more often. You just find yourself doing busywork that isn't all that effective.

You might have read magazines where they tell you that you need to spend two hours in the gym being a bodybuilder to get results. Well, if you want to be a bodybuilder then you can spend two hours in the gym. But as I said, what you find is even a lot of bodybuilders will tell you that all you need is around 45 minutes of *intense* training for optimal results. What tends to happen after you go past the hour mark, is the stress levels from the workout can have an impact on your hormonal levels and your testosterone levels. The workout becomes less efficient after a certain time. If you can do 20 to 40 minutes of focused work you're going to get a lot more out of it than spending twice as long to do the same amount of work. Simply by condensing the time taken, the workout becomes more intense.

You're going to get a much bigger benefit from an intense 20 minutes than you will from working out for two hours. Those long workouts are very draining. It would be counterproductive to you and your business if you're training for two hours a day. You're going to have less time and energy for other things, rather than what we're trying to create here which is a situation where working out gives you more time, more energy, more focus to put into your business, family, and the other parts of life that are important.

I'll tell you a story to show you how effective a 30-minute workout can be. If you're still skeptical about 30-minute workouts, meet one of my former clients Roxy.

Roxy decided she wanted to compete in a fitness show. This was when I was doing competition prep coaching a few years ago. In prepping for her fitness show, Roxy's workouts were only 30 minutes a day. We trained moderately heavy with a mixture of compound and isolation exercises in the gym. We had to go a bit stricter with her diet as she needed to be much leaner than most people would even want to get to if you were to compete (fitness modelling / bodybuilding are extreme sports).

Roxy walked away from that show with two trophies. 2nd place in the bikini category and 5th in fitness. This goes to show that even at an elite level, you don't need to work out for hours to get in great shape, even if that's what you have done in the past. If 30 minutes is enough to get someone a stage-ready physique and two trophies, it's going to be good enough to make some significant changes to your body and health too. Especially if you're new to the gym or haven't been for many years. It's not as big of a commitment as you might think. You can get results in less time than you would imagine.

What should your workout program look like?

A basic, well balanced workout split which includes compound movements for someone who goes to the gym 3 times a week might look something like this...

LOWER BODY - Squats, Lunges, Leg press
UPPER BODY PUSH - Bench press, Dips, Shoulder Press
UPPER BODY PULL - Deadlift, Bent Over Rows, Lat Pulldowns.

You can also go to www.TheMuscleAndHustleMethod.com/man-boobs to get my 'Lose Your Man Boobs' home workout plan.

This of course is a very basic example. There are millions of effective workouts you can find. The most effective workout program is, first the one that you can consistently do and make part of your lifestyle. It needs to maximise efficiency and be simple enough to follow without creating more stress in your life.

If you're going to the gym or doing strength training at home, your workout program should focus on compound movements as shown above. These are exercises that work more than one muscle group at a time. For example, pushups or bench press would work not only your chest muscles but would also work your arms and shoulders. Doing squats will not just work your legs but, engages your entire body. Your core, your back, and all parts of the legs and hips all come into play. If you're doing barbell squats it would work even your shoulders, arms, and traps.

Movements like that, that work your entire body are going to be much more efficient than working on just one muscle group at a time. Again, it is the principle of efficiency. It means you're spending less time in the gym because you're getting more done in the same amount of time by using more efficient exercises.

How do you make working out as effective as possible, when you're spending less time doing it? It's simply making a commitment to focus fully on what you're doing. Don't rest for too long. Do the work and then move on to the next exercise. The aim is to get through the workout, ideally in around half an hour or less. Getting everything done, keeping the tempo high, and not wasting time. Try timing yourself to make sure you're working to a deadline. Don't sit around talking to people, don't spend time watching the TVs. Just get in, get your headphones on, get yourself in the zone, and get the workout done. Cut away all the time wasting, remove distraction and procrastination. Do the work, just like you would in your business.

You're going to feel much better for it afterwards. There's nothing worse than coming out of the gym and feeling like you haven't done anything. Just get in, get it done, and get out. Don't hang around, take whatever rest you need to have a drink, catch your breath, and go again. Choose a suitable weight that's going to challenge you and push through it. The more effort you put into it, the more effective it will be. You get back what you give in the gym. If you're lazily watching the TV's you're not getting much of a workout. Simply being in the gym isn't sufficient – you need to work hard while you're there.

If you don't know how to work out in the gym, or you cannot get to the gym, that is fine. You don't have to go to the gym. Everything you need is within your own body. There are loads of compound exercises which challenge you, and work more than one muscle group, that you can do with just your own body weight. You can still do squats, pushups, pull ups, dips, etc. With a body weight workout, I would tend to rest even less, because you want to keep moving and blitz through it as quickly as possible. Get your heart rate up and the blood pumping.

If you can achieve that via the movements you're doing, that's going to have a positive effect on your mood, it's going to have a positive effect on your body fat levels, it's going to have a positive effect on your muscles, and the way your body looks. It's going to have a positive effect on your all-around energy and drive. Exercise doesn't have to be this perfect workout plan that takes loads of planning and hours of your time. Just pushing your body for 20-30 minutes a few times per week is going to bring the benefits you're looking for. Commit to doing the work and get it done.

If you're really pushed for time; as I said you don't even have to go to the gym. You could, if you really wanted, have a great workout in five or ten minutes. Think of ways to elevate your heart rate, and get you sweating. Even if you're just jumping up and down on the spot; any fully abled person can do that. Often, we limit ourselves because we overthink it. We think that we need to go to the gym or we need to lift weights. That's great and it is the most effective type of training, if you can do it, but if you can't then there is always something that you can do. Doing something will always be better than doing nothing. The most effective training routine, primarily, is the one that you can follow. Everything else is secondary to that. There's no such thing as a bad workout. Start focusing on what you can do, and not what you can't!

Another thing that stops people getting started working out is if they have old injuries or niggles. Even if you have a bad back, you could still go for a ten-minute walk. There's always something you can do. I've seen people with disabilities, missing limbs; they've lost their legs, they've lost an arm, and they still manage to do some kind of activity, and even competing at a high level in a particular sport. If they're not finding excuses, then neither should you. Don't look for reasons you can't do something, but instead focus on what you can do. Make the best of the situation you're presented with.

The action step for this section is to get moving, to start exercising. Get to the gym or do something at home. Shorten your workouts. Try to be more productive with your workouts. Get more done in less time. Train smart and hard, rather than for a long time. Just make sure you're doing some exercise on a consistent basis. Consistency, not perfect, is the key. Make a commitment to doing something at least twice a week from this point forwards. That is a platform you can build upon.

The easiest way to start is to find an activity that you like. Find something that's going to get you a little bit more active, perhaps your favourite sport, or even if it's just walking for 10 minutes. Start small, start with the easiest possible thing that you can do. If you don't have a gym membership that doesn't mean you have to wait until you get one. Just do something that's going to get you moving. Do a little body weight workout or go out for a ten-minute walk. Kick a ball around with your kids. It doesn't have to take up too much time.

If you're not doing anything right now, your fitness levels are probably not going to be in a place where you can do that much. You'll probably find that doing five or ten minutes is going to feel like you've done two hours anyway, depending on your current fitness levels. Just focus on making a start, because the hardest thing to do is start. If you get past that, you're well on your way. If you sit here, think about it, and find reasons not to do it – well like I said – starting is the hardest part.

With that in mind, you want to choose the easiest way to start. You don't want to have any barriers that are going to get in your way. You want to choose the easiest kind of activity you can do and just make a start. I've said this 4-5 times now, because it is so important. Start.

Physical Appearance

In my personal training days when I was in the gym, I'd often walk around and see people in the gym that had been there for years, but their body didn't look trained, their body wasn't changing. They weren't losing weight, they weren't building muscle. Nothing was changing. They'd come in, go through the motions day in, day out; they'd be spending about two hours in the gym and nothing was happening.

One of the things I used to like doing is calling them over and giving them a 15-minute mini-workout. We called them 'wow sessions' back then, to show what we could do as Personal Trainers. I'd give them a 15-minute wow session for free. What we achieved in that 15 minutes felt like more than they'd ever done in all the years that they'd been going to the gym. It just goes to show what you can do in a small amount of time, when you do the right things.

You don't have to be restricted by the gym or what you have around you. As I said there's not really any excuses. You can incorporate more movement, more activity into your daily life. Just little things, it's the little things that add up. For example, taking the stairs instead of the lift, parking your car or jumping off at the station a little bit further away, just so you're walking a little bit more. You don't even have to actively try to exercise. You can exercise without even having to think about it. Just by doing more activity in your day to day life. Every little bit counts.

Building Muscle

Do you want to get the Million Dollar Body that gets younger women's heads turning? What if I told you that you could have that in 12 weeks?

That could happen, depending on where you're starting from. When you're productive and doing the right things, you shortcut the journey to building a great physique. It's like putting your foot on the accelerator and slamming it to the floor, but we do it in a way that's not so drastic that you can't keep going and maintain it over the longer term.

When you go through a physical transformation much changes beyond the number on the scales. Your body shape changes. Your posture changes. Your presence changes. *Who you are* changes.

Think about your posture. You're walking to a board meeting with your chest out, head up, walking with a new confidence and certainty about yourself, which brings with it a presence in the room. It gets heads turning and everyone in the room stops, looks, and listens to you. They want to listen to you because you present yourself as a leader. What kind of physique creates that presence?

A muscular, lean physique creates that presence. Someone with broad shoulders, big chest, someone who looks good in a suit and out of the suit as well. It doesn't matter what you're wearing. You could have the cheapest suit or the cheapest clothes, but they look more expensive when you have that million-dollar body wearing them.

You know what that looks like when you've got broad shoulders, you've got a big chest. You're starting to see an outline of abs rather than a big belly in the mirror. What does a leader of men look like? Is that you now? Close your eyes. Visualise what does a leader of men look like? Ask; how do I become that image?

The best way to become that leader of men image you have in your mind is to start training. Lift weights, compound movements, and follow the diet plans we've gone over earlier in the book. Start going to the gym if you can. Just get to the gym and start strength training. The first step is to get started. Take imperfect action. Everything else will follow from there.

Check out my No More Man Boobs program at www.TheMuscleAndHustleMethod.com/man-boobs.

When I first began my own transformation, I started working out at home. I started doing what I could at home. I did pushups, body weight squats, pull-ups. I had a pull-up bar on my door. I just did what I could, even when I wasn't at the gym.

Back then I was in a place of very low confidence, low self-esteem. I had low self-worth at the time and I thought it was going to be like that forever. I didn't have any confidence with women, I was always a very shy, introverted guy as a kid and to be honest, I still am. I was never the most forthcoming when it came to attracting women or even just speaking to women. Being out of shape compounded this problem.

When I started thinking about getting myself into shape I was more social than I used to be, due to meeting new friends at college and work. I was going out, I was drinking, and I could see my body going the way I didn't want it to go. I was getting a belly, I had man boobs and I really didn't feel good about the way I looked. It was only when I saw the photographs of holiday pictures on the beach that triggered me into starting to take action. I decided that I didn't want to be that person anymore. I got to a point where I said, "Enough is enough. I need to do something about this".

I knew who I wanted to be, and I wasn't being that person at the time. I had my role models, I used to watch WWE wrestling. There were guys on there like Hulk Hogan, Mr. Perfect that had such charisma and character about them. They were big, muscular guys. They were the guys, as kids, we all wanted to be like. "I want to be a wrestler. I want to look like that. I want to have that amount of confidence where everyone's cheering my name". That's where I wanted to get myself to.

You might be reading this at a different stage of your life. You're probably a bit older than I was then, and already successful in other parts of your life. It doesn't matter what age you are, you can still do this. Everyone can make a positive step in the right direction. You don't have to be an athlete or a bodybuilder to do it. You can make progress, simply by starting today. In a week, a month, or a year, you will be in a much better place than you are right now, if you start today.

If you want to make excuses, and procrastinate, that's fine. We all do it in every area of our lives and business. It's just how the brain works. It wants to protect us from potential threat and leaving our comfort zone is perceived as a threat. It always wants to revert us to default, to stick with what we know. We're safe with our current belief patterns and habits. But it's important to become aware when you are doing this, so you can quickly get out of your own way. I have become better at becoming self-aware and getting out of my own way because I have a coach to pull me up on this when I'm doing it. If you want to win big then now's the time to get out of your own way and take imperfect action. Get yourself moving. You must want it; why else would you be reading this book? Put those dreams into reality.

What is the first action? Get yourself in the gym, try a body weight workout. If you can't do any of that just get out for a walk. Find a way of increasing your activity levels. Make a start and let things snowball from there. The first step is the hardest.

If you want to follow one of my workout plans go to www.TheMuscleAndHustleMethod.com/man-boobs.

Systemise

We want to make a healthy lifestyle something that is easy to sustain. Like I've said, you probably don't want to be an athlete or a bodybuilder. You're a busy guy, you have your business, your family, and you want to be fit, healthy, and look great; without it taking over your life.

That's why we want to systemise your fitness, just like you would a business. You can have your body working for you on autopilot when you set up the right systems and routines, that serve your goals and make your life easier. Being fit and healthy doesn't require massive sacrifice on an ongoing basis. It does take some work, and effort, but it serves you and the effort pays itself back many times over. Let's dig into how to systemise your body, to have it serve you on autopilot.

5 EASY SUSTAINABILITY

Build A Body on Autopilot

Why do you want to build a body on autopilot? So you don't have to think about it. We don't want our health and fitness goals to feel like a chore. We want it to come naturally. Just like in your business when you've got things up and running, you can take a little step back and start to systemize things, start to automate some of the processes, to get more staff in to do everyday tasks for you. It's the same for your health and fitness. Habits are like a computer program for your brain. Once it becomes a habit, it becomes programmed or hard wired into your brain and it begins to run on autopilot. You don't have to think about it, it just happens. It becomes part of you and shouldn't feel like it's taken over your life in any way. It's just a small part of your life. You've become someone who is fit and healthy, and will remain that way, without feeling like you're going out of your way or sacrificing a lot of time and energy to do it.

It's important for sustainability that you integrate this into your life. If you feel like you're running on will power and having to motivate yourself all the time, you're going to struggle. Will power has a shelf life. There's only so much discipline and will power you can sustain before it runs out.

You don't want this to be hard. You don't want to feel like you're going too far out of your way when making these changes. You don't want to run on willpower. Instead you want it to feel very natural, to be part of you; a natural part of what you do in your life. This not only makes it easier, but also much more enjoyable.

If you're running on willpower, there's going to be a time when you hit a wall and want to stop. Will power is a finite resource, and there's going to be other – more important – things you need to focus on. You don't want to be running on willpower to make fitness work. It drains your energy and feels like a chore, there's going to be a time when you're going to want to give up. Probably sooner rather than later. This feeds into cycles of low belief, every time you run out of will power and 'fail', it gets psychologically harder to pick yourself back up and try again.

When you are running on willpower it's like doing something you don't want to do. For example, you probably don't want to go to the gym after you've done a long day of work, but you push yourself to do it because you feel like you must. You're tired, you've had a hard day, you're stressed, all you want to do is go home and sleep, or just kick back on the sofa. The willpower part is motivating and pushing yourself to get to the gym and work out. You'll do this for a while, but it feels like an obligation, and nobody likes being obligated to do things they don't enjoy. That's why we're entrepreneurs and we work for ourselves. We want freedom of choice in our lives.

What we want, rather than having to force ourselves out of obligation, is to feel like it's just part of our day. Something that happens on autopilot, without having to motivate yourself to do it. Maybe even something you look forward to, but at the very least something natural that you just do – like getting dressed in the morning.

When you have built the right systems into your lifestyle, it becomes part of your day just like getting up and going to work. With your business, you don't question it, you know it must be done, it's your passion and part of your life. When we wake up in the morning, we don't give ourselves a choice whether we want to go to work today, or you shouldn't be doing anyway. We know we must work, it's just part of our lives if we want to make money and be successful. If we want to live an abundant life, we must work for it. We should be doing the same with our health and body. If we want to build a good quality, healthy life, to live long and prosperous; exercising should just be part of our lifestyle. Your health is more valuable than any amount of money you make in your business, especially when you're comfortable and well beyond worrying about covering your living expenses.

Research suggests that to build a habit it takes about 66 days. At first it will be willpower, the discipline to get started and do what might be uncomfortable, but the more you repeat a task, the easier it becomes. If you go back to one of the best ways of describing a habit, what I like to use as an example is when I was a kid learning to tie my shoelaces. When I was first learning to tie my shoelaces, it would be quite difficult for me. I had to get my mom to show me. I had to practice how to do it repeatedly, and it all felt like a big effort. It was hard work, but obviously, because I've done it so many times, it's now a habit, it become a part of me and not something I need to think about. Indeed, the idea of not being able to tie your shoelaces now is laughable.

Obviously when I wake up in the morning and put my shoes on, while tying my shoelaces, I'm not thinking about *how* to tie my shoelaces. I just do it, it's just programmed into my subconscious brain as a habit. I can get up first thing in the morning, it's 5:30am, I'm tired, haven't fully woken up yet, and I can tie my shoelaces without having to think about it or even look at what I'm doing, because it's a habit and it runs on autopilot.

There are many other examples like this, if you think about it. Learning to walk is another great example. For a toddler learning to walk, it's a lot of effort to them. It's the biggest, most challenging thing they've ever done. They must practice, they have to hold onto things, they will fall and get back up many, many times, but they don't let that failure stop them. They have to keep trying, they have to repeat the process day after day. Now, as adults, we're able to walk without thinking about it. It's not a situation where every step we take we must think about what we are doing, and exert effort to correct ourselves, like we do as toddlers. Again, the idea is laughable to us now. We just walk, and we can even run, without having to think about it. It's become internalised as part of who we are. Totally embedded in our nervous system as a habit that takes place automatically. Getting to this level of mastery is just daily repetition. It's simply using daily success habits. Doing the right things, repeatedly, over time.

Time blocking is a very good strategy that I like to use to make this easier. Protect your time. For you to make this a part of your day, part of your lifestyle, it's important that you book an appointment with yourself like you would for an important meeting. Protect that time and don't let anything disturb the time which is set aside for you. If you block out 30 minutes to do some exercise, that's your appointment with yourself. Trying to keep it at the same time every day is a really good way of building that habit and soon it just becomes part of your day. Eventually, once it's a habit, you're not thinking about it. That's a piece of advice I often give to clients when starting out, "Let's see where we can fit this into your day consistently, then let's protect that time and make it a habit". Where can you find half an hour to book a personal training appointment with yourself?

If you're busy, just start off small. Everyone can find a small amount of time to dedicate to exercise. It often requires less time than you think. If you really wanted to, you can have a great workout in as little as five minutes. Four minutes even. Yes, I've designed 4-minute workouts for some of my busy clients. Four, Five or ten minutes a day is enough if you really are pushed. You don't need a lot of time. Doing 5-10 minutes of intense work beats doing nothing, hands down.

If you struggle to maintain a consistent routine, perhaps you travel a lot or have a lot of unpredictable things come into your diary at work; it's about learning to be adaptable. The only thing you need is yourself. You don't need any equipment, you don't need gyms. You have all the tools you need within yourself. If you think about it, burning calories, all you need to do is elevate your heart rate. You could do that jumping up and down in your hotel room, if you wanted to. If you do that for five minutes, then you would have a pretty good workout. Do 5 minutes of non-stop burpees and tell me that isn't a tough workout. You're not going to get jacked like this, but it will burn calories and improve your fitness. Simply move more.

There's always a solution to a problem, you just have to get a little bit creative and think outside of the box sometimes. A lot of people, especially entrepreneurs who are always juggling their time, have limiting beliefs thinking that to be fit and healthy they've got to go to the gym and spend an hour or more there. Especially if they've done that in the past and been in pretty good shape before. You really don't have to do that. You just need to find small blocks of time and commit to making the best use of that time.

For a lot of people, if they can't make it to the gym for an hour or more, then they end up doing nothing. Even if you were just to jump about for five minutes in your hotel room, or in your office, you could increase your fitness and improve your health. It's not the 'best' workout possible, but it's a lot better than no workout. There's no such thing as a bad workout. The only bad workouts are the ones you don't do. It's all about thinking outside of the box and getting creative to find solutions. Do you want to take control and change your body, or are you ok staying stuck where you are now?

What about healthy eating, how do you make that easier? As long as you focus on eating protein at each meal and getting your portion sizes right, it doesn't always have to be what you might typically think of as 'health food'. If you do want to eat healthy, it's not too difficult. As I said earlier, there's plenty of food around you. You can just grab a meal from the supermarket or a takeaway place that is ready to eat. Just because it is quick and convenient, it doesn't have to be unhealthy. Most supermarkets nowadays have lean, ready cooked meats like chicken breast, fish, etc. already cooked and ready to go. All you need to do is open a packet and eat it. You don't have to worry about cooking or cleaning up. There's coffee shops everywhere. You could get yourself a healthy high protein salad in most coffee shops. There's options for fast food out there, but fast food doesn't mean you have to eat junk food. Simply find healthy options that are quick, simple, and convenient. There's no reason to be helpless and resort to eating junk.

After finding the simple solutions that work for you, we focus on automation. By automation, what we mean is building a habit. Once you've done something for long enough, once you build it into a habit, you do it without thinking about it. It becomes automated in your routine. As I said, protect that time, block it out of your calendar, do it every single day, and soon it becomes a habit. Just like when you brush your teeth. You get up, you go to the bathroom and grab your toothbrush, you're not thinking about it too much, you just do it because it's automatic.

Having that understanding that this doesn't have to be hard is the start. Then gaining the experience of working out in a gym and just getting there consistently is the key. When you have experience under your belt, and you've turned this into a habit, you don't need a fancy new plan to follow, you just go, and you know what to do. You step in the gym, there's not much looking around and thinking, or wasting time, you go in there with a purpose. You know what you're doing. You get in, you get the job done in 30 minutes or less, and you get out.

It's just practice, practice, practice. Repetition is key. It's taking that first step, getting in the gym, and moving forwards. Start by following a plan, start by tracking your food and once you've done that, often enough you get to the point where you can do it without thinking about it. Once you've tracked your food for long enough, you know roughly what portions look like, and what you should be eating. You can estimate it, adjust based on feeling, and do pretty well. This is disastrous if you try and do it to begin with though. You don't have the experience necessary, so you must build that system, build the habit, to make your life easier.

You get yourself to a place where you don't have to track everything anymore. For example, I've prepped for competitions before without even tracking my calories, because I know what I need to do. In fact, I placed 2nd in my first fitness show and I never tracked a thing. I've been doing it for so long I just know roughly how many calories; how much protein, how many carbs, and how much fat there is in every meal I eat. I could prep myself and a client for a competition without having to track or weigh all my foods and still get in very good shape. That's simply because I've practiced for many years. It's the same with the gym, I don't need to follow a workout plan because I've been doing it for a long time. You can get to this stage too, but it comes after learning and following a structured plan for a long period of time to get the basics embedded as habit.

I know that every now and then I might want to try some new exercises, I might want to try a different workout plan, but I don't have to rely on that because I've been doing it for long enough now that I could just go in and workout. I know how to train specific areas of my body and it's just part of my lifestyle at this point. It's what I do, it's who I've become. It's a practice that is simply part of my life.

Like running your business; you're probably at a point now where you could do your job with your eyes closed, but it wasn't like that in the beginning. It probably took years of hustle, putting in the work, consistency, before you could get yourself to that place, it's the same with health and fitness. Put in the work up front, with the view of it becoming a habitual part of who you are.

When I started, I had to build that habit. It was a lot of back and forth; always starting and stopping as my mood shifted. I'd do it for a bit and then I'd stop, I'd fall into old habits. Go back to eating junk and drinking too much. You've got to be prepared to fail at times. That's the only way you're going to learn. What tends to happen, though, is people will 'fail' and they see that as the end point. If you see failure as a learning process, and an opportunity to grow, then you can build upon that. You can learn from your mistakes. If you see it as the end and quit, you're doomed to repeat that cycle forever.

At first, when I was starting out, I was stopping and starting all the time. I started working out at home. I'd do maybe a month of good exercise, and then I'd get bored and give up. I would see results as well, I'd feel the difference, my muscles were filling out, my biceps felt harder; I would see results and then I'd stop. It was like "I've got some results now, I don't need to work as hard". I'd get complacent and end up back where I started. But it was only when I kept going back to it, I kept reading more, I kept learning about nutrition, implementing things, and I started seeing better results which spurred me on. Eventually, it just stuck. I simply never gave up, and through trial and error, managed to find a system that works.

I got myself into the gym. I went to the gym for the first time with a few friends and was quite out of my depth. I felt intimidated because there were all these big guys around me. There was lots of noise around, lots of grunting and the gym rats doing what they do, lifting weights. That really wasn't my environment. I come from a very quiet place. I'm not a loud person, so to put myself into that environment was quite daunting for me at first. It's only when you take yourself out of your comfort zone and you put yourself into a new environment that allows you to experience growth.

I'm a big believer in surrounding yourself with good people, like-minded people who have been on the journey that you want to go on. I'm a big believer in being the small fish in a big pond. If you're a big fish in a small pond, then it's time to go out and get yourself out of your comfort zone if you want to move forwards.

6 GETTING AN R.O.I. FROM THIS

Could building your body help you to make more money and grow your business?

Why is your body important to performance in business? Many reasons. Health, energy, drive, etc. You want your body to be congruent with the business you're running. You want to look the part yourself, as well as presenting – and being - the best in your business.

There's a lack of congruency if you're out of shape. You've got your business to a place of success and hopefully financial freedom. You run your business to a high standard, but you're not presenting yourself at that same standard. If your body is not at a high standard, there's the gap there. It's like you're a six-figure earner, but you're driving around in a Ford Fiesta, when you should be driving a Lamborghini. It doesn't make sense.

That can be a problem because people can see that there's something missing within your business. How can you expect people to trust you, believe in you, believe you can help them, if you can't take care of yourself and present yourself in the right way?

Imagine an opportunity to speak on stage about your business has come your way, but you don't like the way your belly hangs over your belt line, and you can't button up your blazer because it's too tight. There's a worry your trousers might split.

We all know how passionate you are about your business and you could talk all day about it. The problem is, you don't have that confidence in presenting yourself in front of your peers and prospects, so you decide to hide behind your laptop and present an online seminar instead. I hear this all the time from entrepreneurs. Missing opportunity because of self-doubt and uncertainty from not feeling comfortable with how they look. The body you're presenting to the world is very different to the man on the inside. It's certainly not to the high standard you've set in other areas of your life. I know some public speakers who charge $10,000 for an hour on stage. For that kind of money, you wanna be damn sure you're delivering certainty to your audience and not having to worry about your trousers splitting or your belly hanging out.

I've known speakers who are great at what they do, but lack confidence in their own skin and have started to decline public speaking opportunities, because of this. Hiding behind the laptop when the real opportunity and money to be made for you is in the public speaking events could be costing you a fortune. If you're charging $10,000 for a gig, that becomes a very expensive problem.

Let's say you're turning down 2 opportunities a month. That's a $20k a month problem. That becomes a $240k per year problem. That's not including any additional revenue generated off the back of that in products or services. Perhaps you're not playing at that level. Maybe you're just a regular sales guy. But here's the thing, people are all the same. People buy certainty. If you're lacking in certainty, even just slightly, it comes across to your prospects and customers. Even if you sell over the phone or online. People don't have to see you in person to detect that.

It comes across in your tone of voice. If the man you are is not congruent to the man you present to the world, there becomes a lack of certainty, a breakdown in trust. A totally different conversation is subconsciously communicated between you and your prospects. Neither of you will even realise this and it can be as little as a half percent lack in certainty, that is enough to stop your prospects investing in you.

How much money are you leaving on the table?

Being overweight is costing entrepreneurs and companies billions every year. Increasingly companies are realising this and investing in coaching for their staff and providing them with exercise and changing facilities, so that they can improve their health, and get a return on investment from the increased output that brings. It's not just about reducing the amount of sick days as you're probably thinking. A healthy body means a healthy mind. That means more energy and better decision making.
More work done in less time equates to more time, more money, or both. Both of which are highly valuable for you.

Of course, staying overweight will cost you a lot more than money. You'll get a much bigger return on investment from sorting yourself out with improved health, confidence, energy, and get to enjoy more time on this planet. Time, energy, and health are more valuable and precious than any amount of money.

Coming from a Personal Training background; I know it's in the fitness industry, but I've been in the industry a long time and I've seen fat personal trainers who are very good at what they do, very knowledgeable. However, there's an incongruency. Unfortunately, this is a world of first impressions, we are very quick to judge people at first sight. If you're a Personal Trainer and you're out of shape, it doesn't matter how much knowledge you've got. What people see is what they're going to get from you. People will be coming to you because they want to be led by you, they want to be taken on a journey by you, and they want to become the person that you've become. If you're presenting yourself as being overweight, lacking in energy, lacking in drive, lacking in confidence, that comes across to your audience, to your employees, to your customers, and they can always see that. It might not be obvious, but subconsciously they can see it and that can have a negative impact on your business and on how people perceive you.

In the fitness industry, in Personal Training, it's a little bit more obvious. No one wants a fat personal trainer, but it doesn't matter what business you're in, what industry you're in, what kind of business you're running; that same message subconsciously comes across. It's human nature to make judgements on the way other people look. In business, if you're overweight, you're often deemed to be incompetent, even if you're not. There's research that has been done to back this up. It's not politically correct to talk about it these days, but that doesn't stop it happening. If you've got a million-dollar business, don't you want a million-dollar body to match?

You want to be someone who walks into a room and gets the heads turning, drawing attention to your presence immediately. There's a certain feeling and aura about you as you walk into a room. You walk in with your chest out, standing tall and you have a certain presence about you that you're someone who's to be taken seriously, you can be trusted that every word you say is true. You come across as a leader, and people can feel that before they ever hear you say a word.

You'll be glad to know that you can use the same success habits you've used to build your business to transform your body. You've got all the tools already, you just need to repurpose them for this area of your life. You don't need to start again learning a whole new bunch of actions. You're already capable, it just requires a small change of perspective.

How do you do that? Just like you've built your business, you build, you systemize, and you have a long-term vision. Building your body is the same as building your business. You've got to put in the work. You've got to turn up and do the work, you've got to put in the reps in the beginning. In other words, you've got to get the workouts done, you've got to do them consistently.

Then once the business is up and running, you need to systemize and automate things. That is your habits for your health and fitness. This is what makes it sustainable. That will be your habits and the things you do every day that are automatic. You get yourself to a place where working out becomes natural, it becomes part of your lifestyle and is a habit. Eating healthy or eating a well-balanced, moderate diet becomes a lifestyle for you, it becomes a habit where you're not having to think about it. It's systemized. It just happens.

When we talk about vision, ask; in your business, what is your big vision? What is your why? Why are you doing this? What is your purpose? It's the same with your health and fitness. We need to have a bigger 'why'; a reason why we do this. When you look at the big picture here, it's not just to have the six pack abs for a holiday. The big why could be, for example, you want to live a longer, more prosperous life, to see you kids grow up, get married, and have their own kids. You want to have energy to have more drive and focus at work, build a more successful business because you've got a message or a product that you need to get out to the world.

Maybe it's about being more efficient at work. Having more focus and energy so you can do more in less time. What benefits is that going to have for you? It's going to mean you can spend more quality time with your family, you're going to have more energy with your kids, and with your wife. The reason we're doing this is for the bigger picture, the bigger vision. The things that are your highest values in life. How do they align with your physical transformation?

How does getting the body directly lead to you getting this ROI and improving your business? When you've got the body, it gives you a new level of confidence. You will likely close more sales or be a better leader. It's going to give you the fitness to be not just physically fit, but mentally fit. You can have more energy, more drive, more mental focus at work. You're going to be more productive, so you're going to get more done in less time. You can create more time. We all have 24 hours in a day, but you're going to get more done in those 24 hours than your competition. You'll get more done, that's going to allow you to increase your income or scale your business. The biggest sticking point in many small businesses is the energy and focus of the leaders. There is only so much of you to go around. You don't want to crash and burn by midday and have to reach for a coffee and sugar fix to get you through the rest of the day.

You're going to have more mental clarity. You're going to make better decisions in your business. You're able to think fast on your feet and there's going to be a new level of certainty about you. Within your business, that's critical because people buy certainty. People want to feel certainty when they do business with you. If you're uncertain about what you do, what you're selling, if there's a lack of certainty in who you are, people can subconsciously read that about you. Immediately they won't trust you. If you have that certainty, it's going to give you a much higher closing rate and feed back again into a new level of confidence.

The hardest part is starting. It's a little bit of a vicious circle. You work hard, you play hard, when it comes to health and fitness, taking care of yourself; there's not much energy left. To create that energy and increase that capacity, you must get started. As I said repeatedly in this book, the hardest thing is starting, but once you've got that first workout out of the way, the second one is a little bit easier. What you'll find is your energy will increase and you'll get to a point where you do want to go to a gym and do a workout. You do want to work out and you have the energy to do it. Maybe even it doesn't feel good when you miss a workout. The most important thing is that you make a start, you take action today. That is the most important thing to do right now. Don't get caught up in perfectionism about the best thing to do or the ideal this and that, just take the first step.

If you're not sure how you're going to benefit from implementing the things we've talked about thus far, I'll tell you for certain; the best way not to get an ROI from this, is to not do it. I guarantee nothing will change if you do nothing differently. The definition of insanity is doing the same thing over and over and expecting a different outcome, as Einstein once said.

If it just gives you just a little bit more energy to spend with your kids, that's going to be an ROI right there. An ROI doesn't necessarily have to mean a financial gain. An ROI could be more energy to play with your kids without them wearing you out. An ROI could be an improved sex life with your wife, therefore improving your relationship. An ROI could be living a longer happier life. If you achieved even one of these outcomes, would that be worth it to you? A few more years of your life. You're going to see your kids grow up and have grandkids, and you've still got bags of energy to play with them. How much would you pay for that? Let alone getting it for free – maybe even making more money in the process. The best investment you can ever make, where there's a guaranteed ROI, is in yourself. Learn to back yourself. It's the safest bet you'll ever make.

Looking back at your life, think about all the things that you potentially could miss. Treasured moments in your kids' lives because you were too tired or too busy working. Going to school events. Watching them play sports, missing dinner because you're still at the office. Just to be there to see those moments that you never get back.

It's almost a fail-safe formula. You can't do anything but get a positive ROI on this. Your health underpins everything you do. To put it another way; without your health, everything else you do is pointless.

The action plan at this stage is to follow The Muscle & Hustle Method. Start with the build section. The hardest part is building. Once we've got through the build phase, everything else becomes easier. The hardest thing to do is start building the routine, start building the habit. From there it's a practice, just repeat and systemize until it's such an ingrained part of you, it's like getting up and brushing your teeth.

7 SUCCESS HABITS

Win big without even thinking about it. Why is that important? It's important for long-term results. You've probably tried everything else in the past. You've probably tried following plans, and been on diet after diet, and it probably feels like you've seen results and then you can't stick with it. You make progress, then get stuck and before you know it, you're back to square one.

A lot of diets, and a lot of the marketing out there is for a quick fix; but it's not a quick fix that you need. You wouldn't be looking for a quick fix in your business or if you were redecorating your house for example. You don't want temporary solutions, you want security. It's the same for your health and fitness, you don't want a quick fix, because then you'll be forever looking for quick fixes, and there's no such thing as a quick fix. They're just temporary solutions that don't last. The only person who can take control of this is you.

Those that are the most successful play the long game. It's important to build this as a habit and make it part of your lifestyle. It's important for long-term results, it's important for sustainability and it's important to set a high standard for yourself. A standard that matches the standards you've set in your business and other parts of your life. Going back to the incongruency idea, if your body doesn't match the standards of your business, there's a lack of congruency, there's a lack of certainty, there's a lack of confidence and people can see that.

You already have these habits, these abilities within you. You've used them to succeed in other parts of your life. What do you need to do to apply to them to your body?

You have all the tools you'll ever need. All you need to do is repurpose the habits that you've already built, repurposing them and using them on your health and fitness. You've already got the work ethic from business, you just need to apply it to a new area of your life. You've already got the commitment, again you just need to apply it to this new area of your life.

It's not going to take away from your business. Your business is already running, you've already got it out there. You just need to apply the ambition and the drive that made you succeed in business, to a new obsession – your physique and optimising your performance. These are all tools you already have. As I said, you just need to repurpose them and use them in another way. It's the same formula. People who know how to be successful can typically apply that to anything they dedicate themselves to. Success leaves clues.

It's the same process you used to build your business. You built your business by hustling, by putting in the work in the early days. You need to do that with your body and health now and any other goals or aspirations you may have. Set a little bit of time aside for doing it every single day, consistently. It's just consistent small efforts, every day. It doesn't require big efforts, it shouldn't be a chore, it shouldn't take you a lot of time. Just make small, consistent micro-commitments every day, stick with it and you will succeed.

If we look at a big goal, the big vision, you can't just fast forward to the end result of that goal and achieve it overnight. Goals must be broken down and reverse engineered. If you look at what goal you want to achieve over a year, how can we reverse engineer that goal? It must be broken down into smaller monthly goals. What do you need to do each month to achieve your goal in a year? What targets do you need to meet to achieve your monthly goal? We then have to break our monthly goals down into weekly goals. What is your goal for the week? What actions do you need to take daily to reach your weekly goal? When you break it down into small micro-commitments, daily commitments, it turns a big goal into much smaller daily goal, bite size chunks, which make a once daunting goal more attainable.

All you need to do is be consistent with it. Break your goals down into small manageable chunks. It's all about baby steps, one foot forward after the other. As we said earlier, it's like learning to walk. When you were learning to walk as a kid, you had to take one step and then the next step. Maybe you had to hold on to something. You might have fallen over a few times, but you got back up, you tried again, and you learnt to walk. Then you learnt to run. Now the idea of not being able to stay upright is laughable.

Creating the healthy lifestyle and fitness habits is just the same as habits you've used since you were born, from day one. It's the same learning process. It's just the same success formula and habit-building process. You just repeat it again, applied to this area of your life.

Even if you drink, like to eat a burger or you've got a lot of bad habits, you don't need to stop all those habits; you just need to adjust some things. It's not about stopping everything you like doing, even if they are 'bad' habits. It's about learning to work with those habits. We've all got bad habits, even the fittest person in the world has bad habits. I've been in the fitness industry for over 17 years, and I still have bad habits. I still like the odd drink and I still eat some 'naughty' food from time to time, and I want to keep doing those things. I don't want to be living a lifestyle of an athlete all the time, just eating dry turkey and broccoli every day. I want to go out and eat a pizza with my family. I want to go and have a burger. I want to get a take-away at the weekend. I want to have a few drinks with my friends. I will continue to do these things.

Life is for enjoying. You see, the mistake people make, which is why it becomes unsustainable, is they take away all the 'bad' habits which tends to be all the things that they like doing. What they find is they just can't keep that up. If you keep doing what you enjoy doing it's much easier to sustain it. This is what brings results – doing the right things repeatedly, rather than in short little bursts,

If you like going for a drink every now and then, you can still do that. If you like eating take away and eating at nice restaurants, you can still do that, but there must be balance there. It's not something you want to be doing every day. I'm not saying you can live a totally unhealthy lifestyle and expect to get in shape or get healthier. Just that you shouldn't go too far to the other end of the spectrum where you're deprived and miserable. By taking something away, you're going to want it more. Restricting yourself from things you like is a recipe for disaster. It's the child part of our brain kicking in. Think when you tell a kid "No" they want it more and do the opposite of what you tell them. We are no different as adults. Exercising moderations is the way to go.

For example, in January people try and stick to 'dry January' where they don't drink any alcohol for a month. To me it's pointless because what's going to happen in February? They're going to make up for all the drinks they didn't have in January and drink twice the amount in February. It ends up being pointless. If you just drink a moderate amount in January, you don't have to worry about doing a dry January. You just maintain a good, healthy balance and then you won't overdo it in February either.

You don't need to cut out all the things you enjoy doing, even if they are bad habits. Instead make small adjustments and incorporate some new good habits to restore the balance within your lifestyle. Focus on working on one thing at a time. To build a new habit, just work on one thing at a time. If you do feel that you drink too much, then start with reducing your alcohol consumption. It doesn't mean you've got to cut out drinking all together, just reduce it.

A client recently told me that one of his problems was he drinks on average five times a week. On our coaching call, he said, "Ed, I'm going to cut out drinking and see how I get on". I said to him, "Do you enjoy drinking?" He said, "Yes, I do enjoy an occasional drink". I said, "Why are you going to cut that out? Why are you going to restrict and punish yourself? You don't have to cut out drinking. Why don't we just try reducing it a little bit?".

He took his drinking, which was five times a week, and reduced it to three times a week. That's a healthy positive step in the right direction, and we're not taking away something he likes doing, so we get the best of both worlds. He gets to have a drink, and he gets to lose a bit of weight at the same time, because we're taking away some calories. This could be potentially 500 to 1000 calories a week in those two extra days that he was drinking. Little changes like that will make a huge difference. You don't have to cut anything out, just apply sensible moderation and be aware of what you're doing. Find where you have leverage to make positive changes without significantly upheaving your lifestyle.

Rachel was a client of mine who I prepared for a physique competition. Obviously, when you prepare for a competition, it can be a little more extreme and is maybe perhaps not so sustainable, but we got her into great shape. She's not been able to maintain the level of discipline and deprivation required to stay in competition shape (nobody could), but she has been able to maintain a great physique compared to the shape she was in before she got into fitness. It became a habit for her, she loved it, she stuck with it. Since then she developed such a passion for it that she got into the fitness industry herself and became a Personal Trainer. She had an extra income source from following what became her passion. It all started with a couple of small changes to her lifestyle, and everything snowballed from there.

The journey of a success story starts by taking the first step and then each individual next step, one step at a time. Here's a couple of simple habits you could try implementing each week.

- ✓ Make one healthy change to your diet or lifestyle.
- ✓ Make a commitment to do just a little more exercise/activity than you did last week.

If you implement these simple steps over 12 weeks, that's 24 steps. That could be enough to completely transform your body and give you the platform you need to go on to greater things.

This is a story from another female client I've coached. Over the course of us working together Dolly went from being overweight to doing a fitness photo shoot, and the physical transformation spilt over into other areas of her life, allowing her to excel in her career and relationships.

Dolly was unhappy with how her life was going, prior to us working together. She was self-conscious and not being the person she wanted and knew she could be. This was having a negative impact on her relationship at the time with a partner she'd been with for 9 years. She wasn't going out socially because she wasn't happy or confident with who she was. She would try any fad diet going, looking for a quick result. It was a vicious circle of trying and failing, getting angry about her situation, and then turning to food for comfort.

"Ed changed my relationship with food. I didn't have to go on a drastic diet like I had with previous trainers. I was expecting a diet plan of the exact foods to eat and when. Instead he told me you don't have to stop eating what you like to get the results you want.

What I like about working with Ed is he's not just about fitness and nutrition, we'd talk about parts of my life that had nothing to do with fitness, and it was working on these areas that I found I got the most benefit from Ed's program.

Before working with Ed, I never felt confident putting myself forward for business opportunities and bigger roles. I recently interviewed for a promotion and I got the position. That's something I would have never have gone for before working with Ed".

Vision

This final section of the book is about having a larger vision for your body, and your life. In the previous section I touched on having a greater vision. Here we are going to flesh that out, go into more detail and find a strong 'why' that will pull you towards a better vision for your future. This is where the hard work you do upfront can be multiplied and come to pay itself back multiple times over with improvements across all areas of your life.

When coaching my clients, this is ultimately where the focus ends up. Initially it is about weight loss, building muscle, feeling better; but in the end it's about creating a more abundant life and having a bigger impact in business, having more self-confidence, better relationships, being a role model for your children, and all the other big picture things that we value.

8 YOUR BODY IS YOUR BIGGEST ASSET

The reason you would want to do this is so that you've got the competitive edge and you can outwork the competition. As we said earlier, having the body, you're not only going to look good and have that confidence, you're going to have more energy, more drive, more focus. You're going to increase your capacity to do more. You'll be getting done more in your 24 hours than the competition.

You've got to focus on implementing the success habits and just backing yourself to take the risk. You've backed yourself in the past, you've taken risks. It's backing yourself to follow the same process. If you follow the process, you can't fail. That's all you need to do. Have that resilience, that assurance, that certainty that "this is going to work, if I follow the Muscle & Hustle Method". The safest bet you'll ever make is when you back yourself.

You can make your body your biggest asset through continued self-development. You've already invested in yourself with your business. You'll need to continue investing in yourself further if you want continual growth. Not just financially, but with your time and by putting in the work. By doing it, committing, and taking action to create the future you want.

You're an action taker. You wouldn't be where you are now if you weren't. It's simply about applying that same mentality, that same winning mentality that you already have, to your health, to your body, and to yourself. It all starts with you and your body. That's where I started. If I didn't transform my body, I'm certain my life would probably look very different now. I would not have the business I have. I probably wouldn't have been in the coaching industry. How can I help others if I couldn't take care of myself? I probably would not have met my partner either.

My life would have taken a very different path. Without what I've achieved in my health and body, and taking care of myself first, that wouldn't have allowed everything else that's fallen into place to happen. I would still be stuck. Stuck where I was all those years ago.

You've got to stop thinking and start doing. You can think about it for as long as you want and you're not going to get anywhere. If you just take imperfect action, you'll make more progress than if you take no action at all. There's two possible outcomes from taking imperfect action. You either WIN or LEARN. You can't lose so you may as well back yourself. I'll say it again, it's the safest bet you'll ever make!

Being A Leader and A Role Model

A story of leadership from my good friend Richard. Me and Richard started working out together back in my early days of Personal Training. I had maybe 2 or 3 years' experience in the gym at the time and Richard was just starting out. He followed my lead and just did what I did, not just in the gym, but outside of it too. He followed my way of eating and the lifestyle I was living. Doing this he started to get great results and transform his body quickly.

This was back in the day when I was into bodybuilding and that was the lifestyle we were living. Training hard and eating chunks of protein every 3 hours. This was before we had kids and a business to run of course. We had plenty of time to dedicate to bodybuilding. It was the discipline that fitness provided us with, and the speed of change that inspired Rich to apply the same principles to other areas of his life. What are those same principles?

"Consistency of action", he said. "If you want to achieve some kind change, transformation, or reach a goal it requires consistent action towards that goal. If you want to 'master' something you can't just dabble. You have to go all in".

We were going all in at the time with our training. That's why we got the results that we did. We were fully committed to doing what needed doing. I always say it was my early days in the gym transforming myself, and fitness in general, that was a platform for me to go on to greater things. It's where I first began taking control of my life and growing towards something better.

More recently Richard has used that 'certainty of outcome' that he now possesses, as a result of our time training together and 'consistency of action' and has applied it in his life by leaving a good 9-5 office job for something greater by starting his own business. He can live life on his own terms and see his two young kids grow up because he has much more flexibility and freedom in his schedule.

He said, "part of my decision was inspired by you, Ed, and what I've seen you do with your life. The fact that you're constantly adapting and growing, and you never let things go stale".

I love the fact that I'm able to lead and inspire others and add massive value to someone's life which will filter down through the generations into our children's lives, and their children. What we do now is meaningful, and I'm proud to inspire my friends to bigger and better things.

Have you ever had that feeling when someone walks into a room and you can tell that they're important, even though you don't know them. There's a certain presence and aura around them, as they walk into the room. That's the kind of impact you can make, by presenting yourself in the right way to the world.

You want to be a leader because you want to get more of what you want in life. You want to help others at the same time get what they want in their lives. You want to lead by example. You want to be a role model for your family and a superhero to your kids.

You want to be the dad that everyone else's kids look forward to playing with when they come over to your house. You've got the energy, you've got the time to interact and play with the kids. You don't want your kids looking forward to going around to your mate's house, because he's more fun than you are. You want to be that guy that everyone wants to be around. This includes your colleagues, family, friends, and your children.

A leader is someone who leads by example. Like attracts like. You attract the people into your world that you are most alike. If you want to attract leaders into your life, you need to be a leader yourself. You need to be the client that you want to attract. If you want people to invest in you and invest at the highest level with you, you need to be prepared to invest at the highest level in yourself. You can't expect others to do things that you're not prepared to do yourself. I don't just mean financially, but with your time, effort, energy, belief, and desire.

You do that by showing up in the world every day and putting your money where your mouth is. Taking action and doing as you would expect others to do. Leading by example. My clients wouldn't want to come to me to be led on a journey if I haven't been on that journey myself. People want to be led by someone that has already walked the walk. That has been on the journey that you want to go on. People want to be led by someone who will take them to the promise land and get them to get there quicker, to shortcut the process to their success.

You might be asking, "who are you leading by example when I'm changing my body?". I'm leading other men that want to look like me. They want to experience some of the success I've experienced in transforming my body. Some of the success I've experienced in my business that can be attributed back to transforming my body. That's the kind of person that I would attract into my world. Because I've done it myself, I'm doing it now. I'm growing. People want to grow with you. You can do the same thing.

It's fine if you're not an outgoing extraverted guy either. People will still follow your lead if you have that presence that comes from self-mastery. I'm not an extraverted guy. Often the guys that talk less and listen more are the best leaders of all. They listen, they understand, and they get where you're coming from. People that spend a lot of time talking, they talk a good game, but they don't always walk the walk. They're just good at talking and that's about it. You can silently lead by example and create a powerful impact on the people around you through setting the right example.

How do we set the right example? We need to set bigger goals. Set new goals that are ten times bigger than your current reality. To create that vision. Paint a picture of it. What does it look like? If you could change the world, what would you do?

Then start breaking those goals down into yearly, monthly, weekly, and daily action steps. Action steps to implement today. Be consistent with achieving these daily goals. Take consistent daily action. Just the same as any other goal, only this time we're looking to take much bigger actions. Having developed more confidence through our physical transformation, we can re-write what is possible for us to achieve.

Set these big goals and start with conquering your body. You'll develop the belief and drive to take over the world. When you achieve the goal in your body, it gives you confidence, it gives you that certainty and you believe that you can take over the world. Not literally, but you have that feeling of assurance and certainty about you. That's a good place to be. That's what we strive for. That carries over to other parts of our lives.

The reason we do anything, the reason we're working, the reason we're trying to become the best we can be, is ultimately so we can be happy. To be content with ourselves, and our impact in the world. To be able to look back in old age, without and regrets about opportunities missed, or things we wish we had done. To provide a great life for our family and loved ones. How are you moving towards that today?

It's important to keep moving forward with new goals because satisfaction has a shelf life. When we achieve our goals, it's quickly a question of "what's next?". We get there, we're happy, we've made it, but then that happiness very quickly diminishes. It's important that we continue to set goals and keep ourselves moving forward towards the next thing. Especially as entrepreneurs, we're always in motion. We're living in a fast-paced world. Our lives are very fast-paced, we always want to keep growing and moving forward. If we're stuck, then we're not happy with where we are.

At the same time, it's important to be grateful and appreciate what we already have. Appreciate and enjoy the journey, because if you're constantly striving for the next big thing, with the assumption that it will bring you happiness; you're never going to be happy. There will always be the next thing to strive for. It is important to strive for more, of course, but it's also important to be grateful for what you have. That will hopefully include a body that serves you. Good health, lots of energy, and a physique that inspires. When you get that balance right, that is the place you want to be. That is happiness.

Using *The Muscle and Hustle Method* we've talked about in this book, we're just applying those same habits to other areas of your life. We've talked about how you have already applied it in your business, and we've talked about how you can apply it with your body and health. Now ask, how can you apply it to the rest of your life? Building good relationships with your friends and family, for example.

It's the same success formula that you can use in all areas of your life, to keep growing. Once we've reached where we want to be in a certain area, you have to ask, where else do I want to go?

If we've got the business we want, and we're happy with where we're at; we've got the body, what's next? Is it to spend more time with your family? Is it to travel more? Life is a long journey. There's so much we can do to enjoy life and appreciate every moment. What does that look like for you? What other areas can you apply this same formula to? To keep yourself growing, to keep yourself moving forwards?

Simply go back to the drawing board. Write down your vision and your big goals. I can't emphasize enough the power of writing down your goals. Goals are much more powerful when you write them down and you can see them in black and white, as opposed to just keeping them in your head. Writing them down allows you to get them out of her your head and really focus on them, and even helps create a neurological pathway in your brain. Write down your big goal, your big vision. Break it down into smaller chunks. Break it down into even smaller chunks until you're down into micro commitments and small baby action steps that you can start taking today.

Consistency is key and breaking it down into these baby steps ensures you don't get overwhelmed with the size of the task ahead. A goal without a plan is just a wish. Now you have the process, and the body to build even greater things upon. Go forth and do it.

I was a very shy kid, didn't have much confidence in myself. My first goal was to change that. I thought the best way I could change that was through changing my body. My initial goal was to transform myself. I applied these methods, which didn't come naturally to me at first, because I hadn't really, at that time, achieved anything. The only thing I was relying on was my goal and my vision for a better future. Writing it down and moving towards it, refusing to quit. I had the knowledge that this is what I want to achieve, and it took many years of trial and error to get myself there.

That was a learning process along the way. That's a process that I can now carry over to other areas of my life. The ability and the discipline to transform your body has so many benefits. The discipline to succeed in transforming your body crosses over into so many other areas of your life.

I used those same skills to become a Personal Trainer. That was never something I imagined doing when I was younger. I had no real vision of what I wanted to do, to be honest. I wasn't a sporty kid. The last thing I thought I would be is a Personal Trainer or be part of the fitness industry. I was last to be picked for the sports team at school. I didn't enjoy sports, I wasn't strong in any way, I had nothing about me that would indicate that I would be some kind of fitness professional. For me to end up in that industry was purely a creation of the vision for the life that I wanted. Anything is possible if you want it, and you work for it.

Often, we can't see what the big vision is until we work with someone who has already been on the journey and they can see what we can't. Going back to surrounding yourself with people that have been there, who have done it, who have been on the journey that you want to go on. That's why I love coaching and I also love being coached. My coach has a vision of the journey that I'm on, that even I can't see yet. For me transforming my body was the leverage point to bigger and better things. It was the catalyst.

It allowed me to build a business in the fitness industry, where I can work for myself, I can help others. I can pull others through from where I was, to the place where I am now. Pull them through the same journey that I've been on. Onwards and upwards to a better life.

Having this vision and taking my life to the next level has allowed me the confidence to meet my fiancé. It was always an ambition of mine to have a family. For a long time when I lacked confidence and was too shy to speak to women, I wondered if it would ever happen. I've now done that. I've got a beautiful fiancé and a young son. These are all things I was having doubts about at first, when I was shy and out of shape. I didn't see how it was possible for the person I was at that time to achieve that.

You must be resilient and persist with the process. I followed the bumpy journey, and here we are today. It's a journey and it's about appreciating what you've got. I appreciate where I am right now. I've managed to do all the things I've done. I've got a healthy son, a family. I'm very grateful for all of this. There's still more that I'm striving for, though. I'm always looking for the next big thing to pursue. At the same time, I'm in a place where I'm content, I'm happy. That if everything was taken away, I've still got my family, my son, and that's why we do what we do.

One of my favourite activities is to create a vision book or board. A board is better because you can see it on the wall. Find pictures of what you want out of life and stick them on your vision board/book. It could be pictures of your dream home, your dream body, your dream car, your family life, travel destinations etc.
This might seem a bit out there but just be open minded and give it a go. Everything you've ever achieved always started with an idea and a picture in your head. By cutting out pictures and looking at them every day, you create strong neurological pathways in your brain that help you in achieving those goals.

9 CONCLUSION

You're almost ready to go out and start implementing *The Muscle & Hustle Method* to achieve amazing results in every area of your life. Remember, to get the best results, you must start by working on yourself first. You are the driving force, the engine behind everything you do.

You must apply *The Muscle & Hustle Method* to your own body and health for your engine to run efficiently and at full speed, rather than misfiring and chugging along. So you can perform at your very best in all areas of your life. You can use the same success habits that took you from start up to six-figures and repurpose them to create a 'Million Dollar Body'. You already have all the tools you need. Once you look and feel great, and are performing at your best, you can use *The Muscle & Hustle Method* and re-apply it your business once again to take your profits from six figures to seven. What other dreams and aspirations do you have? How can you apply *The Muscle & Hustle Method* to these areas? The only limiting factors are the ones you place on yourself. So, get out of your own way and go make it happen.

Follow each of the three steps of *The Muscle & Hustle Method.*

1) Build - You built a successful business by putting in the work. To achieve great things takes hard work. There's no two ways about it. Now is the time to put in the effort to building your body and health. Nothing comes easy. If it were easy, everyone would do it. But you can make it easier by having a plan. What's the big goal? Write it down and reverse engineer it into small daily goals and take consistent action every day to reach those goals.

2) Systemise - Once you find a winning formula, rinse, and repeat until it becomes a habit. You can probably do your job with your eyes closed now. That's because you've consistently repeated daily tasks for such a length of time that it has now become a habit. There are probably elements of your business that you've been able to systemise. Perhaps by hiring staff, getting a PA, or using technology to automate things, meaning you can free up some of your time while your business still runs efficiently. We want to achieve this level of mastery with your health and fitness, and in any goals you may have, so that it becomes hardwired into your brain. It becomes part of who you are, and just happens without you having to think about it.

3) Vision - Once you've gained mastery, what's next? Where else can you apply *The Muscle & Hustle Method?* As highly driven individuals there's always going to be a big vision. If you're anything like me, you're never satisfied. There is always going to be a new project on the horizon, more work to be done, improvements to be made. The day we stop will be the day they're nailing the coffin shut and throwing dirt on us.

With that said, with all our drive and passion to be the best, we must also adopt a mindset of contentedness. Of gratitude. To stop and look around, appreciate what we have and how far we've come on this journey we call life. If you always want, want, want, you will never be happy. Without gratitude, we miss all the amazing things that are already in our lives.

I get that you're driven, and you're working all the hours God sends to make a better life for you and your family. Just stop and take a few minutes out of your busy day to give your kids some love and attention when they want it. That's worth more to them than any amount of money you will ever make. Tell your wife you love her and take her for dinner from time to time. Even get away for a romantic weekend. Make some time for yourself and switch off so you can work on your own development, and health.

Appreciate and enjoy what and who you have in your life in the here and now, rather than always focusing on the future. The years will soon pass you by. Years you can't get back.

When we can strike the perfect balance of drive and gratitude, that's where the magic happens!

It's a great place to be. A place of true happiness.

Congratulations! You've made it to the end of the book. That shows me you're in the 10% of guys who take action and are committed to following through. So, what's next?

Next Steps

If you've enjoyed reading this it's time to take action and implement what you've learnt. Without implementation, it's just information… and information is useless without implementation. Sometimes we just need some accountability to follow through and keep us on the right track. If you're anything like me and my clients, you want to take the quickest and easiest path possible, because your time is precious.

If you'd like to find out about working with me personally, to have certainty that you're on the quick and easy path go to www.EdDjafer.com. I do take on 1-2 new clients per month if it's a good fit for both of us.

You can also reach me via Facebook at www.Facebook.com/Ed.Djafer. Simply add me as a friend and say "hi".

To your success…

Ed Djafer

ABOUT THE AUTHOR

Ed Djafer is a health and performance coach who loves helping entrepreneurs to succeed in their health, performance, and business.

Ed went from being an introverted, unconfident guy, feeling trapped in his overweight body and engineering job; to transforming himself to having the confidence to step on stage against some of the best men's physique competitors in the world, build a successful business, and become one of the UK's best performance coaches.

You can connect with Ed at www.EdDjafer.com.

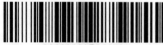

39688382R00051

Printed in Poland
by Amazon Fulfillment
Poland Sp. z o.o., Wrocław